T5-AFY-380

Improving
Your Health
with
Vitamin A

by Ruth Adams
and
Frank Murray

Preventive Health
Library
Series

Larchmont Books
New York

NOTICE: This book is meant as an informational guide for the prevention of disease. For conditions of ill-health, we recommend that you see a physician, psychiatrist or other professional licensed to treat disease. These days, many medical practitioners are discovering that a strong nutritional program supports and fortifies whatever therapy they may use, as well as effectively preventing a recurrence of the illness.

First printing: June, 1978

IMPROVING YOUR HEALTH WITH VITAMIN A

Copyright © Larchmont Books, 1978

ISBN 0-915962-24-1

All rights reserved. No part of this book may be reproduced without permission in writing from the publishers.

Printed in the United States of America

LARCHMONT BOOKS
6 East 43rd Street
New York, N.Y. 10017
212-949-0800

Contents

CHAPTER 1

Your Need
for Vitamin A

THE TRAGEDY OF nutritional ignorance on a worldwide scale is highlighted in an article from the *New York Post* for June 13, 1977 on the prevalence of blindness in many Eastern countries. It is estimated that as many as 11 million children under the age of six in developing countries of the world are threatened with blindness for simple lack of vitamin A, which is present in many inexpensive foods readily available in their communities. But their families do not know of the risk of blindness from lack of vitamin A, so they do not feed their young children with the fruits and leafy vegetables that would supply enough of this fat-soluble vitamin to prevent blindness.

More than one million children in India suffer from *xerophthalmia*, which brings blindness and another 20 or 30 million have severe eye disorders as a result of not getting enough vitamin A in their food. **Just a capsule of this vitamin given every few months would remedy this lack, for vitamin A is stored in the liver and doled out to body cells as need arises.**

In the United States, the U. S. Senate Committee on Nutrition and Related Human Needs listened in shocked silence as Dr. Arnold E. Schaefer, who was then chief of the Nutritional Program, Division of Chronic Disease Programs of the Public Health Service, spelled out the results of a survey of the nutritional state of Americans. The findings were almost beyond belief. We are accustomed to hearing of malnutrition and hunger in the poor, disadvantaged parts of the world, but it is alarming indeed to hear that conditions in our own country—among rich and poor alike—are as bad, and in some cases worse, than in many poverty-stricken nations.

In the case of vitamin A alone, **the survey found that 13 per cent of everyone examined had less than acceptable levels of the vitamin.** It also uncovered eight cases with eye symptoms indicating a drastic deficiency of vitamin A.

In a survey released February 26, 1968, the U. S. Department of Agriculture discovered that **20 per cent of the American population is eating a nutritionally poor diet.** Almost one-half of the households in each region of the United States surveyed had diets that failed to meet the recommended allowances for all nutrients as established by the Food and Nutrition Board of the National Academy of Sciences, National Research Council. **As for vitamin A, approximately one-fourth of the people surveyed were deficient.** Projecting the USDA figures into the entire American population, we find that perhaps 40 to 50 million Americans may lack the amounts of vitamin A which experts believe they should have to be well nourished.

A survey on levels of vitamin A in human tissues was done in 1969 and reported in the March, 1972 issue of *The American Journal of Clinical Nutrition.* This is a professional journal for doctors, nutrition experts and university professors who teach biology and nutrition. The four authors of the study are Army medical personnel and Ph.D.'s.

They performed autopsies on 372 bodies, some of whom had died accidentally, some from diseases of various kinds. They were from five widely separated parts of the country:

Missouri, Iowa, Ohio, Texas and California. In one of the localities the researchers also tested for pesticide accumulations in the liver, since there is some evidence that certain pesticides deplete the body of vitamin A. Their tests included upper income people as well as very poor people. There seemed to be little difference in the results, so apparently having enough money to buy vitamin A-rich foods or supplements has nothing to do with the results obtained.

Their conclusions were as follows: "It appears that, depending upon unknown regional influences liver **vitamin A stores may be low in 12 to 37 per cent of the five population groups studied.** The 12 to 37 per cent figure is in agreement with recent studies from Canada and New York City. Comparable values have also been published from the United States National Nutrition Survey.... The agreement between the data obtained in this study and the studies cited suggests that the population groups of the study may be typical regarding vitamin A nutriture. Further studies are required to define more precisely the magnitude of the problem of vitamin A insufficiency and whether it is the result of nutritional or other factors."

In other words, this official study showed, as have three or four other studies done in recent years, that **up to 37 per cent (more than one-third) of all Americans are probably not getting enough vitamin A to provide their bodies with the amount they need for optimum health.** Or to put it another way, from 20 to 30 per cent of our entire population is probably in the "poor risk" group regarding vitamin A nutriture.

An even more shocking revelation comes from a Canadian survey, which was reported by Dr. T. Keith Murray to a nutrition congress held in August, 1968 in Puerto Rico. Dr. Murray discussed 100 autopsy specimens from each of five Canadian cities (500 people in all), of which **more than 30 per cent of the individuals had less than 40 micrograms of vitamin A per gram of liver.**

"This is less than the level they were born with and the

newborn of any species is notoriously easy to deplete of its vitamin A reserves," Dr. Murray said.

Eight of the specimens in Ottawa showed no stores of vitamin A at all. In Montreal, 20 per cent of those examined had no vitamin A stores either.

The ages of the individuals studied ranged from stillborn infants to people 92 years old. Most of the subjects were over 50. People who died of various diseases seemed, generally, to have less vitamin A stores than those who died in accidents. But there apparently was no relation between the nature of the diseases and the amount of vitamin A that was found. The average Canadian, like the average American, is thought by health authorities to be getting about five times the minimum required amount of vitamin A in his daily diet.

"It is hard to blame diet alone," Dr. Murray said. "Even allowing for wastage, cooking losses and uneven distribution, it does not seem likely that so many of our population do not get enough vitamin A to maintain their reserves."

It is believed by Canadian experts that the condition they found may not necessarily be the result of poor eating habits, but may instead come about because of the things in our environment which deplete our stores of vitamin A or which cause us to use it at a faster rate than we can get it from our food. Pesticides were incriminated. The researchers then looked into the drugs those Canadians had taken before they died, but could find no relation between any given drug or drugs and the store of vitamin A in the liver. They were especially interested in drugs which reduce cholesterol, for cholesterol is a fatty substance and, as you know, vitamin A is a fat-soluble vitamin. Such drugs might, they thought, interfere with the body's use of vitamin A, since their purpose is to block the action of the fatty substance, cholesterol. They could find no apparent tie between drugs and vitamin A storage.

Then they took up the amount and kind of fat in the diet. They studied the level of vitamin E in the diet, since this is apparently related to the way the body uses vitamin A. They looked into the amount of protein these people had been eating, for the amount of protein in the diet is linked, too, with the way the body uses vitamin A. On diets low in protein, vitamin A is not used very effectively by the human body. But it did not appear that lack of protein was the answer, although some of the older people might have been eating less than the recommended amount of protein.

Dr. Murray explained that it is not easy to alter the absorption and utilization pattern of vitamin A so it must be something as yet undiscovered which is robbing people of the amount of vitamin A which they need. Perhaps, he said, it is some combination of poor diet and something in our environment—pesticides?—that does the damage.

Is vitamin A important? Must you have it to be healthy? Must you have it every day? These are some of the questions we will be answering in this book. Another nagging question: Can you get too much?

Briefly, vitamin A is in charge of the good health of all cells that line anything in your body. This means not just linings that you can see—like the lining of your throat and nose—but also the linings of the digestive tract, respiratory tract, genital tract, the prostate gland, the eyes, the blood vessels, etc. Many cancers begin when cells apparently go haywire.

In addition, **vitamin A is essential for the formation and preservation of sound teeth and bones**. It also plays an important part in normal vision. Eyes are exposed to light all day. Light uses up a substance in the retina of the eye—visual purple. A good supply of vitamin A must be on hand to restore this substance by the next morning; otherwise, you may find it difficult to see in dim light. This condition is called "night blindness."

As we will see, **vitamin A is important in maintaining a healthy skin,** in possibly preventing or alleviating acne, in protecting you against air pollution, in impeding aging, etc.

One of the first symptoms of vitamin A deficiency may be not only an inability to see in dim light, but also

a great sensitivity to glare. After that you may notice trouble with the lining of the nose and throat. Your doctor may discover that the linings of other organs are atrophied (wasting away), then horny. You then become more susceptible to infections, since these cells are partly responsible for protecting you against germs. Further, vitamin A maintains the health of the mucous membranes. It regulates cartilage for bone development. It is involved in the production of an essential substance in the adrenal glands which are involved in protecting us from stress.

The best food source of vitamin A is liver, which may contain as much as 76,000 International Units in a serving. Fish liver oil is the basis for most vitamin A food supplements. All green and yellow fruits and vegetables are rich in vitamin A, for it has a yellow color. Carrots, spinach, beet greens, apricots, peaches, kale, tomatoes all contain plenty of vitamin A.

Of course, if you want to be scientifically exact, you have to admit that vitamin A as such doesn't exist in carrots or in any other vegetable or fruit. The chemical substance known as vitamin A exists only in food products from animal sources. But all green and yellow fruits and vegetables contain a substance—carotene—which is made into vitamin A in your body.

Although you may be getting enough vitamin A in your diet, there is a chance that you may not be getting and absorbing all of the vitamin that you need. You could, therefore, be suffering from a partial deficiency that keeps you from being as healthy as you might be. **Since vitamin A is fat soluble, certain conditions of the body may hamper absorption:** liver damage, for example, or impaired absorption of food from the intestines. Lack of certain digestive juices, illness, the presence of certain substances which destroy the vitamin, cooking and frying foods at high temperatures—all make the vitamin less available to the human body. You may be deficient in vitamin A if you have been taking mineral oil for some time, because this laxative is extremely destructive of vitamin A. Also, chronic diarrhea, celiac disease or a badly functioning gall bladder or pancreas can also interfere with absorption.

There is some loss of vitamin A, or carotene, when you are preparing meals. Though the heat needed for cooking does not destroy the vitamin, it is rather easily destroyed by oxidation, suggesting that you should keep cooking utensils covered at all times. Since vitamin A is not a water-soluble vitamin, it is not destroyed by soaking or exposure to light as some of the B vitamins and vitamin C are.

You should make every effort to get plenty of vitamin A-rich and carotene-rich foods at mealtimes. As added insurance, food supplements are suggested. The best and most dependable source of vitamin A in a food supplement is fish liver oil, which is available in a tasteless, odorless form quite different from the nauseating cod liver oil preparations earlier generations had to take. Your health food store has many vitamin A supplements and preparations.

Most of you already know the value of raw foods and realize that we should eat some raw foods at every meal. However, in the case of carotene, the fibrous cells of the fruit or vegetable must be thoroughly broken down before the carotene is available to the body. This means either chopping, cooking, chewing very thoroughly or juicing. Such foods as peaches and tomatoes do not need much chewing obviously, but carrots and some salad greens may be hard for some people to assimilate all the carotene in the food. There are also products made of carrot oil. These are, of course, quite high in carotene and are the perfect vitamin A supplement for vegetarians.

According to official standards, healthy adults need 5,000 units (International Units) of vitamin A daily. For children, the recommended daily intake varies from 1,500 units for infants to 4,500 for boys and girls up to 12. Pregnant women need 6,000 units per day, and women breast-feeding an infant need 8,000 units each day.

Some newspaper columnists writing on health make a lot

of fuss about your getting too much vitamin A, So does the American Medical Association. And the Food and Drug Administration tried unsuccessfully to prohibit the over-the-

Vitamin A Is...

Fat-soluble, meaning it is stored in the body, so that it is not essential to provide vitamin A every single day.

Responsible for the health of the retina of the eye, the production of visual purple in the eye, which helps us to see at night, the maintenance of skin and linings of all body openings and organs, resistance to infections, bone development, maintenance of the myelin and membranes of our bodies, maintenance of color vision and peripheral (side) vision, maintenance of the adrenal gland and synthesis of certain hormones.

Present in most abundance in liver, kidney, carrots, spinach and all other dark green, leafy vegetables and yellow vegetables and fruits such as apricots, peaches, nectarines, yellow squash, sweet potatoes, butter, egg yolk.

Not to be taken in excess. Taking very large amounts of vitamin A over long periods of time can produce unpleasant and dangerous symptoms, which, in adults, disappear when the vitamin is withdrawn, but which may persist in infants and children.

Destroyed in the body by mineral oil laxatives, by several chemicals, estrogens and other drugs.

Required officially in amounts of 5,000 International Units by adults, somewhat less in children, depending on age.

Available in capsules up to 25,000 International Units.

Safe in amounts up to 20,000 units daily.

counter sale of vitamin A above 10,000 I.U. Warning against taking vitamin pills without a doctor's prescription, they would have you believe that almost anyone who buys food supplements on his own is risking grave danger of overdosage of vitamin A.

The important thing to remember is to read the labels and not to take massive doses of vitamin A without your doctor's orders. There have been a few cases of overdoses in medical history. By this we mean 100,000 units or more per day. In virtually every case, these people disregarded the suggested dosage on the labels. Mothers gave their children concentrated vitamin A by the tablespoon as they would have given cod liver oil, rather than by the drop as the label suggested. In one recorded case, some arctic fisherman went on a fish liver-eating binge in which each man got something like 1,000,000 units of vitamin A. But to use such isolated incidents as a basis for warning against too much vitamin A is ridiculous.

CHAPTER 2

Protecting
Your Lungs

"VITAMINS APPEAR TO PLAY a much more vital role in safeguarding lungs from the ravages of air pollution than has been generally realized," reports an article in *Chemical and Engineering News* for June 29, 1970. At a symposium on pollution and lung biochemistry at Battelle-Northwest Institute, a scientist from Massachusetts Institute of Technology told of his experiments with rats in which he found that the two fat-soluble vitamins—A and E—play an important role in protecting lung tissues from harm that may be done by two components of air pollution, ozone and nitrogen dioxide.

These two pollutants are among the most destructive compounds we have loosed on city dwellers from industrial pollution and the exhaust from automobiles that jam our city streets. Certain fatty substances in the lungs are broken down by the pollutants releasing other substances that are highly dangerous. Vitamin E appears to "quench" these substances, rendering them harmless.

Scientists from Battelle-Northwest have been conducting a series of nutrition experiments in which they fed rats a specially prepared diet that was high in polyunsaturates—the fatty substance which is attacked by the air pollutants. Some of the animals got food that contained no vitamin E. Others ate the same diet, supplemented with vitamin E.

The rats were then exposed to a stream of air containing one part per million of ozone. They soon showed signs of severe stress in breathing, and died. **Those which were getting the vitamin E lived twice as long in the ozone polluted atmosphere.** In other experiments, researchers autopsied the rats after they had been exposed to nitrogen dioxide. The animals that had eaten the diet deficient in vitamin E had far less of the polyunsaturates in their lungs than the rats which had plenty of vitamin E. Apparently, the vitamin had preserved the valuable polyunsaturates and prevented their destruction.

Dr. Daniel B. Menzel of Battelle's nutrition and food technology section believes that vitamin E might perform still another beneficial function in safeguarding vitamin A from being destroyed by the air pollutants. "This itself would be an important function," says the article, "because it is now becoming increasingly evident that vitamin A is crucial for the healthy metabolism and growth of epithelial cells." These are cells in the skin and lining of body cavities like the lungs.

At Massachusetts Institute of Technology, scientists have been experimenting with vitamin A, giving it to rats, then examining their lung cells. **The rats which had plenty of vitamin A showed a healthy condition of the lungs.** Those which had a deficiency showed cells that were thick, scaly and hard, instead of being soft and covered with healthful mucus. After identifying a certain compound present in the healthy lungs and absent in the deficient ones, the M.I.T. researchers found furthermore that, when they gave supplements of vitamin A to the deficient rats, this beneficial compound was formed in their lungs within 18 hours, even though they had been eating a deficient diet for a long time.

The researchers went on to say that we know now that **vitamin A can prevent the formation of cells that later turn into cancer cells.** They don't know exactly how the vitamin does this, but they are investigating the process. And now they are wondering whether massive doses of vitamin A may be able to reverse the growth of certain kinds of cancers. We explore this supposition in more detail in the chapter on cancer.

CHAPTER 3

Defending Yourself from Pollution with Vitamins and Minerals

"IT HAPPENS every hour of the day, every day of your life. Dozens, hundreds of drugs, carcinogens and other potentially hazardous environmental chemicals bombard you. Your major defenses against these compounds are enzymes located in the portals of the body—skin, blood, lungs, liver and kidneys. These enzymes break down (metabolize) foreign compounds so that they can be excreted from the body and hence not build up and cause toxic effects."

These are the opening words of an excellent article on how diet can protect from poisons. Written by Joan Arehart-Treichel, it appeared in the July 19, 1975 issue of *Science News*. She was reporting on a meeting of top experts in this field—the Federation of American Sciences for Experimental Biology. Specialists gathered at the meeting came to the conclusion that **one's diet is more important for controlling the unhealthful effects of drugs, for** example, than any other mechanism such as the reactic \ of one drug or another.

It s \s that some people lack the enzymes necessary for handl \rtain drugs. This is the reason they suffer toxic effec... \hen, too, the more drugs and other chemicals the body has to deal with at that moment, the more toxic the effects are likely to be. It seems to us that the same thing must be true of other toxic materials in our environment—pesticides, industrial chemicals, air and water pollutants, cosmetics and so on.

The one single most important food element involved in this protective shield against harm from poisons is protein. As long ago as 1952, a toxicologist reported that a deficiency in protein increases the toxicity of drugs to which people are exposed. Since then lots of other researchers have shown the same thing. Getting not enough protein at daily meals decreases the ability of the enzymes involved to protect against foreign chemicals and drugs.

In one experiment rats were put on a diet deficient in protein, then exposed to pesticides. Another group of rats which were getting plenty of protein were exposed to the same poisons. The pesticides were 2,000 times more toxic to the low-protein rats than those getting enough protein. It seems that the protein keeps the enzymes "primed for action."

If we were living in Eden, breathing only the purest of air and drinking the purest of water, if we could get food totally uncontaminated with chemicals of any kind, if it were possible for us to avoid, every day, any exposure to any toxic substances, we might be able to get along on far less protein than is needed to provide for protection against all these threats from a technological society. But since it is well known now that dietary protein gives protection against all these contaminants, it is wise to get as much protein as we can, since there is no evidence that we can get too much. **Protein food has a built-in guarantee that you will not overeat.**

A second food element which appears to protect us against environmental poisons is a certain kind of fat—the kind found most abundantly in food of vegetable origin—unsaturated fat. A University of Georgia researcher fed corn oil to rats who were then given drugs. Their bodies disposed of the drugs harmlessly in less time than it took for animals who were not getting the unsaturated fat of this oil. **It seems that unsaturated fats play a major role in keeping up the health and efficiency of the enzymes whose job is to protect us from poisons.**

The other food elements involved in this struggle are vitamins and minerals, mostly vitamin A and Vitamin C, and minerals such as zinc, magnesium, copper and calcium. Several toxicologists from Ottawa, Canada reported on their work along these lines. They do not know, they say, just how the vitamins and minerals bring about this protection but they do. A diet which is adequate in vitamins and minerals is much more likely to keep the relevant enzymes in top condition.

One researcher reported the unhappy circumstance which he uncovered in laboratory work. It is possible, said O. N. Miller of the LaRoche Research Center, that sometimes these same enzymes are capable of taking a fairly innocuous chemical and turning it into a cancer-causing substance. So to defend oneself against these poisons it might seem better to eat less of the protective elements. But, of course, this would invite damage from all the other hazardous substances in our environment.

"The message that emerges from the food-drug metabolism research," says *Science News*, "is that a diet adequate in proteins, unsaturated fats, vitamins and minerals is the best way to keep your microsomal enzymes in prime condition to detoxify toxic compounds. The message is a crucial one, since all of us are bombarded with an array of self-imposed, physician-imposed and environment-imposed chemicals, and we need all the preventives against their toxic effects that we can get."

The previously mentioned M.I.T. researchers were working with Dr. Umberto Saffiotti of the National Cancer Institute, who has already proved that vitamin A, given orally to hamsters, can completely prevent the cancers that would normally appear when the animals are exposed to certain cancer-causing substances in our environment.

Over 12 years ago, the National Cancer Institute reported that **vitamin A protected animals against stomach and reproductive tract cancer.** Those animals which were getting quite large amounts of the vitamin showed no cancers when exposed to cancer-causing chemicals.

Dr. Daniel B. Menzel, previously mentioned, noted that the laboratory tests to which the laboratory rats were subjected simulated smog concentrations like those found over Los Angeles or Tokyo on a bad day. The rats which had not received vitamin E died within an average of eight days of continuous exposure to the air containing 1 ppm of ozone. Said Dr. Menzel: "Los Angeles has recorded up to 0.9 parts per million of ozone on a bad day."

Foul air, according to Dr. Menzel, causes an "oxidative breakdown" of the lung, which he compared to butter becoming rancid. "Just as when a bubblegum balloon has a weak point it will rupture at that point, so will the tiny air sacs in the lung."

Dr. Menzel believes that the ultimate solution must be to rid our environment of pollution. In the meantime, however, the Battelle discovery "may ameliorate what is one of the most rapidly rising disease syndromes in the world's urban areas."

There is no way for society to avoid paying for pollution, reports a booklet, *Pollution and Your Health*, available from the U. S. Environmental Protection Agency, Office of Public Affairs (A-107), Washington, D. C. 20460. "If we do not pay for prevention, we pay in other ways—in lost recreational uses of rivers and beaches, in higher treatment costs for drinking water, in damage to crops, forests and buildings and, most importantly, through higher medical bills, time lost because of illness, human suffering and premature deaths." The booklet goes on to say:

"The Department of Health, Education and Welfare puts the total national health bill at about $120 billion a year, most of it for cure rather than prevention. Yet there is an increasing body of evidence and an impressive array of expert opinion that we may be approaching the whole question of human health from the wrong side—that, as a matter of national policy as well as personal practice, an ounce of prevention may well be worth a pound of cure.

"In the United States the once dreaded infectious diseases are controlled through sanitation, immunization and antibiotics. Today we are plagued with chronic diseases that an increasing number of health experts believe are largely caused by environmental factors—where we work or live, our habits, diets or life-styles. The more sophisticated and sensitive our monitoring devices become, the more data we accumulate on the health effects of pollutants and other agents in the environment, the worse things look.

"The battle against diseases must increasingly be fought, not simply in the hospitals and doctors' offices, but in our streets, homes and workplaces; in our air and water; in our food and products; and in our habits and lifestyles. Such a shift in emphasis will require a searching re-examination and radical revision of our popular understanding of, and our public approach to, health care and disease. If environmental disease is becoming "the disease of the century," as it appears to be, then environmental protection must become the most important ingredient in any national health program.

"While much is already known about the health effects of some pollutants, pollution's total impact is difficult to measure. What each pollutant does to a human depends on the physical and chemical properties of the pollutant; the length, intensity and method of exposure; and an individual's ability to tolerate the pollutant . . . virtually all forms of pollution harm people somehow. Some people are especially susceptible to attack, notably the very young, the old, and those weakened by disease. Since resistance to pollution is an individual trait governed by such factors as age, heredity, general health, climate, occupation, residence, smoking and dietary habits, it is extremely difficult to assess precisely the general effects upon a large population.

"Dirty air makes eyes water, burns throats and stifles lungs. Fumes of sulfur and nitrogen oxides, sulfuric acid and photochemical oxidants irritate the respiratory system causing coughing, chest discomfort and impaired breathing. When small particles are breathed in along with these fumes, the irritation—and injury—may increase substantially. Carbon monoxide interferes with the ability of blood cells to carry oxygen. **Heart and nerve tissues are particularly susceptible to oxygen deficiency**, so that carbon monoxide pollution can seriously impair coronary (heart) and central nervous system functions. . . . The total number of such pollutants commonly found throughout the country is not known, but every year thousands of new chemicals are introduced into manufacturing processes alone. It is impossible to discuss the potential health effects of all likely pollutants. . . .

"Like air, water is not limitless, nor free, nor somehow immune to the pollution which affects other aspects of our environment. . . . A 1970 survey of 969 public water supply systems disclosed that 56 per cent had facility deficiencies relating to equipment design, construction or plant condition; 77 per cent of the plant operators were inadequately trained in microbiology and 46 per cent were deficient in the chemistry relating to their assignments; and 79 per cent of the systems had not been inspected by State or county authorities during the preceding year.

"**Sources of water pollution are innumerable.** Major sources can be found in nearly every kind of industrial, municipal or agricultural operation. There are thousands of toxic chemical compounds in use today and new chemicals are being developed every year. Chemical contaminants such

22

as phosphates, nitrates, pesticides, detergents, trace amounts of metals, acid from mine drainage, cyanide, phenols, radioactive substances, solvents and hydrocarbons are all products of our technological society and potential threats to our water sources... small quantities of organic chemicals are present in public water supply systems throughout the country. Some of these are suspected cancer-causing chemicals.... Water that corrodes pipes causes metals to be swallowed by people drinking the water. Comparatively little is known about the effect on human health of ingesting these metals....

"Beyond the physical waste, **environmental pollution may have a more profound effect on man; on mental health,** for example. Most lead poisoning causes behavioral difficulties, perceptual disabilities and emotional instability. Mercury poisoning causes emotional instability, tremors, fatigue, dizziness, memory and speech difficulties and headaches. Carbon monoxide poisoning causes apathy, psychological tiredness, headaches, temporal-spatial disorientation, retardation and psychosis. Psychological impairment following exposure to pesticides has been discussed elsewhere, and a number of studies have linked excessive noise to higher mental hospital admissions, as well as to other psychological disturbances....

"We all receive radiation from natural sources over which we have little control. Our remaining exposure comes from medical and dental X-ray machines; fallout from weapons testing; uranium mines, mills and fabrication plants; nuclear power generating and fuel-reprocessing installations; and various electronic devices... we know very little about the long-term effects of repeated exposure to radiation at low levels. One major hazard is damage to or alteration of human genes, since natural background radiation is believed to be one of the causes of natural radiation mutation. It is generally accepted that any amount of radiation, however small, can cause damage to genetic cells and hence cause an indeterminate number of undesirable mutations. Such

23

genetic damage is believed to be cumulative. Also, it is generally accepted that an increase in radiation exposure can cause increases in the frequency of many cancers," the booklet reports.

"Eager Breathers" is the name of a club in the Washington, D. C. area, sponsored by the Lung Association there. Its members are people who find that when air pollution gets bad their eyes get runny, they suffer from coughs and headaches, they feel depressed and they have difficulty concentrating. Sitting in a room where others are smoking is a form of torture for them.

Some of them have progressed through the series of breathing problems which accompany pollution until they must now spend a certain amount of every day breathing oxygen from a tank. According to one member, quoted in *Environmental Action* for June 4, 1977, bronchitis irritates the cilia, the fine, hair-like appendages that line the lung's air passages. In time the bronchitis becomes worse and the cilia can no longer function. This leads to emphysema, which is today almost a national epidemic. In emphysema the alveoli are injured. These are the tiny air sacs which fill the lungs where carbon dioxide in the blood is exchanged for oxygen.

Once the alveoli have lost their ability to perform this exchange, all parts of the body suffer for all body cells need oxygen. And, according to a Washington nurse specializing in pulmonary and respiratory cases, **"During air pollution periods, you are less able to process oxygen through your lungs and into the blood.** That's particularly true for people with respiratory problems. Carbon dioxide builds up in the blood and that causes the depressed feeling." She says that the high level of pollution in Washington air "causes increases in chronic bronchitis; it sends many asthmatics into spasm; it puts emphysematics into real danger."

According to the National Heart and Lung Institute, "the initiation of environmental lung disease as a result of air pollution in childhood may be the starting point for continuation and progression of such disease in later life." It seems that low level air pollution (not a pollution alert—but just the average day-to-day smog) brings great harm to the lungs of children, accounting for probably half of all acute childhood illnesses.

Low level air pollution may cause infant death during the first year of life. It may increase the incidence and severity of respiratory disease in children. It may aggravate the asthmatic conditions of those millions of American children who suffer from asthma and it may eventually lead to chronic bronchitis.

Officials at the Environmental Protection Agency fear we are making almost no progress in fighting air pollution. One spokesman says we are in danger of falling back to conditions worse than those which existed before we supposedly started to clean up the air. Remember Pittsburgh? And Los Angeles? Says *Environmental Action*, car pollution is the worst offender and as fast as government sets new standards for curbing car pollution more cars are on the road, so the new standards accomplish little.

But other air pollution sources are also doing us in very rapidly. One Gary, Indiana teacher described the symptoms he and his family suffered when the wind was coming a certain way from the steel mills: dizziness, nausea, headaches, burning eyes, inexplicable hunger pangs and tingling pains in hands and feet, lethargy, inability to concentrate on reading or to maintain a train of thought.

"There is no escape from air pollution anywhere in the East," says *Environmental Action*. Plumes of pollution from industries can and do pollute for miles around. St. Louis pollution shows up 100 miles away at levels exceeding federal standards. Big industry threatens economic disaster every time air pollution standards are mentioned.

"There's a great deal of talk about relaxing clean air standards in order to help solve the energy crisis. The argument goes: How can we justify spending money to make the air more pleasant when we have serious problems of energy supply to deal with?" writes Polly Bradley in the

"Most of this talk misses the entire point of the clean air standards: Public Health. Air pollution is a public health problem. It is not an aesthetic problem.

"Air pollution isn't just a middle-class concern. Air pollution, in fact, does the most harm to those least able to fight it—the poor, the sick, the black, the old, the very young, the people who live in the inner core of big cities.

"According to the American Public Health Association," she continues, "**21 million people are 'at risk' from air pollution**. Urban dwellers and industrial workers encounter the most pollution, but many categories of people are particularly susceptible to air pollution. Major factors in susceptibility include:

"Aging or debilitation (weakness).

"Preschool age (when detoxifying enzyme mechanisms have not yet matured).

"Overcrowded living conditions.

"Malnutrition.

"Genetic defects such as asthma, sickle cell anemia, atrial or ventricular wall defects.

"Developmental defects including coronary insufficiency, rheumatic heart disease, chronic bronchitis and emphysema.

"Cigarette smoking or exposure to cigarette smoke.

"Other suspected causes of increased susceptibility are childhood infections, heavy physical exertion and obesity. It is estimated that the conversion of 46 power plants in the eastern corridor from oil to coal (now being considered) could increase the death rate from respiratory and cardiovascular diseases by as much as 40 per cent, unless adequate measures are taken to control stack emissions.

"Of course, these are only statistics. They don't seem real—until I or my loved ones are hit with them. Who wants to become a statistic? Let's have less talk of relaxing clean air standards and more thought about how to go about doing a job that needs doing: making the air clean for everyone," she reports.

So what can you do? First, you must get away from the pollution if at all possible. This is often difficult if you live or work in a congested area. Don't smoke and avoid places where you will be exposed to tobacco smoke. Insist on no smoking where you work. You'll find lots of coworkers are on your side. Don't go to meetings, conventions, parties where people will be smoking and indicate your reasons in your refusal to attend. Lots of people feel the same way.

Support every clean air and/or air pollution measure, local, state or federal, that comes along. Write your elected officials expressing your concern. Join groups fighting air pollution, such as the American Lung Association, 1740 Broadway, New York City 10019, and the National Clean Air Coalition at 620 C Streets, S.E., Washington, D. C. 20003. Avoid traffic jams and superhighways and expressways where pollution piles up as cars proliferate. Move away from sources of industrial and auto pollution if you can. Eat in restaurants that have no-smoking rooms. Ask for the "no smoking" section on airplanes, although this is usually a sham. We have yet to fly in a no-smoking section where there weren't people smoking.

What about diet? First, see that you are getting ample protein. There are two basic kinds of protein—that from food of animal origin and that from food of plant origin. In the first group are meat, fish, poultry, eggs and dairy products. In the second group are all those high-protein vegetarian foods which your health food store can supply: legumes (beans, peas, soybeans, peanuts), wholegrain cereals like wheat, rye, rice, barley, millet and buckwheat. But remember that the wholegrain ones are the only kind recommended. The refined and processed kinds have been so depleted of protein as well as most other nutrients that they do not qualify as recommended foods. Other excellent vegetarian protein foods are nuts and seeds of all kinds: sunflower and squash seeds, popcorn, almonds, sesame seed, pumpkin seed, etc.

Well, then, what else must a good diet have to qualify as a

protective screen against toxic chemicals? Unsaturated fats. These are most abundant in the foods mentioned above—the high protein vegetarian foods. Eating them at meals provides the unsaturated fats. We also make from them the salad oils (safflower, sunflower, corn, and so on) which are concentrated sources of the unsaturated fats and vitamin E as well.

It should come as no surprise to discover that the foods mentioned above are also the very best sources of all the vitamins and minerals with the exception of vitamins A and C, which are, generally speaking, most plentiful in fresh fruits and vegetables, especially the bright green and bright yellow ones. So a diet consisting of nothing but the foods mentioned here—including fresh fruits and vegetables—is the best possible diet to eat.

You will note we have omitted some common foods which line most of the shelves in the supermarket—highly processed cereals, bakery goods, desserts of all kinds, soft drinks and other beverages which contribute nothing to good health, "convenience" foods, candy, chewing gum, snack foods except for the healthful ones like unsalted nuts and seeds.

Not many of us eat diets that are so well planned as this. We cheat a little on desserts. We take candy and soft drinks if they are offered to us. We kid ourselves into believing that some special kind of white bread is so delicious that it must be highly nutritious. Or we are involved in so many activities that we just don't have time to prepare and eat the kind of meals we should.

For people like this, the only answer is food supplements—high-protein supplements and supplements of vitamins and minerals. Brewers yeast and wheat germ are two excellent high-protein foods. Add them to every appropriate dish. Stir the yeast into milk or fruit drinks. Use wheat germ as a breakfast cereal. Include it in every casserole, every piece of baked goods you make.

Vitamin and mineral supplements are available in great variety at your health food store. The fat-soluble vitamins—

A, E and D—are stored to a great degree in the body. Vitamin C and the B complex are water-soluble and any excess is excreted within about four hours. So it's best to take them every day and, if you are taking large doses of vitamin C, space them throughout the day so that you keep your cells and tissues saturated with this very helpful vitamin.

As we have seen in this book, **scientists have found that they can prevent damage from some kinds of urban pollution with fairly large doses of vitamin A and vitamin E.** It wasn't just imagination, because the subjects of the experiments were laboratory rats. Those exposed to the elements of urban air pollution suffered from many of the same symptoms city dwellers experience, including lung cancer. And those which got, in advance of exposure, large doses of vitamin A and vitamin E, in addition to their usual excellent diet, escaped most of the damage. Some of them suffered not at all.

We recommend that you take vitamin A regularly, in addition to eating lots of vitamin A-rich foods like carrots, leafy greens and liver.

We also recommend that you make vitamin E (alpha tocopherol) a regular part of your food supplement program.

CHAPTER 4

Let's Talk About Your Eyes

WHEN HUMAN BEINGS first appeared on Planet Earth, there were no books, no ledgers, no television sets, no microscopes, no telephone directories. There was no need for eyes to accommodate themselves to close work. So our eyes developed over the ages for seeing things at a great distance. The eyes of early hunters searched hillsides and forests for signs of game animals. Their families hunted berries and fruits, nuts, roots, insects and bird's eggs and later planted and cultivated cereal grains.

All of these occupations required far-sightedness. When reading and writing developed (a very short time ago, speaking in terms of human life on earth), we suddenly had to learn to focus our eyes on very close work and keep them focused this way for long periods of time. It was not an easy adjustment to make. Undoubtedly our eyes have suffered from it. One way to help prevent eye strain from close work is to relieve the eye muscles by looking up very often and resting your eyes on something far away—a tree, a building, a cloud, before you go back to close work again.

Our eyes, which are among the most complex and delicate organs of our bodies, must be nourished by the

food which we eat. There is no way for them to get such nourishment except from our meals.

Many aspects of life in a modern technological society combine to make things more and more difficult for those of us who want to remain healthy.

Often the source of these difficulties is so remote and obscure that no one, literally, in all the vast scientific empire has as yet done any research on it. Take light, for instance. Until perhaps 75 years ago, human beings lived with about the same amount of light the animals have. Generally speaking, they got up at dawn and went to bed when darkness fell.

The artificial light they had from candles, oil or gas lamps was hardly more than a dim pool of twilight in the corner of a room, compared with the glare of modern electric lights from which there is no excape for the city dweller, who knows no such thing as absolute darkness any more. Everywhere he goes at night, his eyes are exposed to glare.

There is no indication that human eyes were ever meant to be exposed to this amount and degree of light for so long a time every day. The mechanisms our bodies have for dealing with light are equipped to deal with the amount of light we would get outdoors from dawn to dusk— no longer.

Almost no one, literally, has delved into this problem to hazard a guess as to what immeasurable or slight amount of damage we may be doing to our health just by constantly exposing ourselves for many hours every day to bright, bright light. What has this to do with vitamin A? Listen!

The American Automobile Association published an article on the incidence of driving accidents at night. **It seems that the fatal accident rate is two and one half times greater at night than in the daytime.** Say the AAA authorities on traffic engineering and safety. "Increased attention should be given to night vision, which involves greatly different seeing tasks than day vision.... In the U.S.A. over half of pedestrian fatalities occur in hours of darkness."

The authorities went on to enumerate reasons for the failure of drivers to see as well at night as during the daytime. They say that there are great individual differences in ability to see, both day and night. But since the things involved in the two kinds of driving are so different, the eye test which is usually given during licensing of drivers is not a good test of the driver's ability to see at night.

There are three special hazards to nighttime driving. First, it is just plain harder to see details at night, that is, harder to distinguish objects from their background. Then night driving is made more hazardous because the driver is faced with glare from the headlights of an oncoming car. Finally, after the car has passed, the eyes must recover from the effects of the glare, before the driver sees well again.

Some people see quite well at night. Others are almost blind. Some people are bothered very little by the glare of oncoming cars and require only a few seconds to recover good vision after the car has passed. Burton W. Marsh and Earl Allgaier, the AAA experts, tell us that people who have difficulty seeing at night, difficulty in facing glare or in recovering from glare should be very careful about driving at night. They should drive slowly, hug the right side of the road and be extremely cautious.

They go on to tell us that exposure to very bright light during the day decreases one's ability to see at night. If you spend the day at the beach, without sun glasses, chances are you will have considerable trouble seeing on the drive home. Then, too, they tell us that ability to see at night decreases much more rapidly with age than visual acuity does.

After the age of 20, the amount of light just to see an object roughly doubles for each three years of increase in age. So a person of 33 needs about twice the amount of light just to see a dimly lit object as does a person of 20. At 46, the amount of light needed is again doubled. So the older person should avoid driving at night if possible.

Lack of oxygen can also increase the sensitivity of

the eye to light. Smoking creates lack of oxygen, because the carbon dioxide given off by the cigarette smoke replaces oxygen. So don't smoke while you are driving, especially at night. High altitudes also decrease one's supply of oxygen.

Finally—and these writers got to the most important point last—**vitamin A deficiency causes what is called "night blindness" and sensitivity to glare**. "This generally is not a problem in normal diets," say these authors. "If an individual has trouble with night vision and suspects that this vitamin deficiency may be involved, he should take vitamin A or include food in his diet which has a high vitamin A content."

These authors are not physicians. They are safety experts. But they have obviously consulted physicians who have told them that "normal diets" contain plenty of vitamin A, so we don't need to worry about that in dealing with night driving. But everything the authors have described in this article has to do precisely with vitamin A deficiency.

"One of the hazards of night driving even for the most experienced motorist is dazzle from oncoming vehicles," says *New Scientist* for December 13, 1962. **"The presence of visual purple . . . in the retina (of the eye) is essential for vision at night."** Visual purple is a pigment which is essential for protecting our eyes against glare and allowing us to see in darkness and near-darkness.

Visual purple is bleached out by light—either sunlight or artificial light. The eye regenerates it during darkness. In order for this process to take place, there must be enough vitamin A or carotene available.

Being blinded by the lights of an oncoming car indicates night blindness. Another indication is the inability to adjust to sudden darkness after light. When you go into a darkened theater from a lighted street, how long does it take for your eyes to become accustomed enough to the darkness for you to find a seat? It should take no more than a few minutes. If you step out of your lighted house at night, how long does it take you to be able to see trees, walks, street signs? It should take no more than a few seconds.

Living creatures other than man which are equipped to carry on their activities by day go to bed with dusk and get up at dawn. Since the invention of electric lights, human beings have tended to stay up later and later, using the hours of darkness as if they were really daylight. Hence more and more of this valuable essential substance, visual purple, is destroyed while we watch television, go to late parties or read at night.

One way you can be sure of saving up visual purple is probably to get plenty of sleep at night and avoid any late hours under artificial light. Most of us can't arrange our lives this way, however, so the next best thing—and it's a good idea for other reasons as well—is to get plenty of vitamin A in our diets and diet supplements.

Chlorophyll is that substance in green leaves which captures the sun's energy. Without chlorophyll there could be no life on earth, for all living creatures, including human beings, depend on the food from green plants, chiefly the carbohydrates manufactured by chlorophyll in the green leaves. The process of making chlorophyll is called photosynthesis by scientists. This means creation by light. Only in daylight can this process take place.

Scientists have been studying this rather mysterious process for many years and thought they knew just about everything they needed to know about it. But, according to *The New York Times* for March 15, 1976, they uncovered an astonishing new fact about the whole process that staggered them. It seems there is another compound in the world which can also take the sun's power and convert it into usable energy. This substance is the bacterial form of "visual purple," which, as we have seen, is in the retina of the eye and is essential for sight.

The implications of the new finding that visual purple can also convert the sun's energy into energy useful to man are staggering in many ways. Scientists are now talking about using this substance (in its bacterial form) to create energy

34

for many purposes. Perhaps it can be stored in battery cells and used to fuel cars or heat homes. The prospects are almost limitless, it seems. The *Times* says, "Whether this discovery turns out to be useful or not, it must still inspire awe as one more indication of how much more splendidly complex the miraculous world of nature is than earlier generations could even imagine."

Now that we have established the elemental importance of visual purple (it ranks with chlorophyll as one of the basic materials essential to life on the planet!) we should make note of some related things. First, visual purple reacts with light. It is apparently destroyed or "used up" by light, so that it must be renewed in darkness. New York researchers have discovered, using rats as subjects, that animals given no vitamin A could manufacture enough visual purple to see well if they were kept in darkness all the time.

Other rats, subjected to some light, then darkness, and deprived of all vitamin A, could not manufacture visual purple, but lost it continuously from their retinas. Presumably if the animals had been kept without vitamin A and with recurring light and darkness, they would eventually have become blind if the experiment had continued long enough.

You may think you are getting enough vitamin A. You eat carrots sometimes and have tossed salad often for dinner. But a survey of 151 medical students at Boston University Medical School revealed that 55 of them had night blindness because of vitamin A deficiency. The 55 ate in restaurants oftener, they had less money to spend on food, and they had fewer meals per day than the students with no night blindness problem.

The story of one student is told in *This Week* magazine for September 12, 1965. For several years he had noticed that his eyesight after dark was getting worse. Driving at night, he could barely see road signs, pedestrians or the edge of the road. When he went to the movies he had to wait for fifteen minutes before his eyes had adjusted to the dark so that he could find a seat. He had also noticed a dry skin and itchy eyes, both symptoms of vitamin A deficiency.

What did he eat? We imagine his diet is fairly typical of many college students who have absolutely no idea of the rules of good nutrition. He had coffee and doughnuts for breakfast, hamburgers, dessert and coffee for lunch, lean meat, white potatoes, white bread, dessert and coffee for dinner. When he ate vegetables, they were either beans, corn or peas.

His daily vitamin A intake was about 1,000 units. The official daily requirement is 5,000. He was given 25,000 units of vitamin A in fish liver capsules and was told to add to his diet: milk, ice cream, butter, cheese, liver, fresh fruit, spinach, raw carrots, squash, sweet potatoes and prunes.

Within ten days his night blindness was greatly improved, within two months it was completely normal. And his other symptoms of vitamin A deficiency had disappeared. Many people on reducing diets may run into the same kind of trouble, if they are attempting to reduce on black coffee, lean meat and salads, with little or no fat.

Every official survey of the way Americans eat has shown that lack of vitamin A is very common. Many of us are probably not getting enough vitamin A to protect our health. If, in addition, we are getting far too few hours of darkness to renew the visual purple in our retinas, might these two things not be a significant reason for many of our eye problems?

Aside from its function in helping to make visual purple, vitamin A performs many other helpful biological tasks, as we are learning in this book. It helps to maintain a healthy skin and takes care of the welfare of the linings of things— the lining of throat, esophagus, stomach, intestines, reproductive organs, mouth and so on. It helps us to resist infections. It is active in developing bones and teeth and keeping them healthy. It also helps maintain the myelin sheaths of the nerves which are disordered in multiple sclerosis and polio. It helps us to see colors. It is essential for

36

the healthy functioning of the adrenal glands and the hormones they make.

That's quite a lot of work for one vitamin. And scientists say they are still in the dark as to just how most of these functions are performed. The one thing they know surely about vitamin A is its importance in maintaining our supply of visual purple in the retina of the eye.

There are a number of conditions in which you may have difficulty in absorbing vitamin A from your food. A damaged liver cannot store it. Colon trouble which causes excessive excretion of fats may also cause vitamin A to be excreted, since it is fat soluble. Taking mineral oil and several other laxatives renders vitamin A less available for use. Exposure to a number of antagonists of vitamin A may prevent its absorption. Some of these are sodium benzoate (a chemical preservative used in many foods which the Food and Drug Administration has pronounced perfectly safe), bromobenzine, citral (a flavoring agent used in hundreds of foods), estrogen (the female hormone used in The Pill) and thyroxine, the thyroid gland hormone, when it is present in large concentrations, as when it is given as a drug.

As we know, vitamin A as such does not exist in vegetables and fruits. They contain carotene which must be made into vitamin A inside our bodies. Diabetics may have trouble making this conversion of carotene to vitamin A. The carotene may also be lost if fibrous foods like raw carrots are not chewed enough before they are swallowed. The cells of these tough vegetables must be completely broken down before the carotene is liberated. This is one reason why cooking may help absorption of carotene in the case of carrots and tough salad greens.

Vitamin A as such does appear in some foods of animal origin: liver, eggs, butter and cream chiefly. Many people have been told by their doctors to shun such foods because of their cholesterol content. This would deprive them of much of the vitamin A they should normally have.

So there seem to be many sound reasons for taking

vitamin A supplements. And check the vitamin A chart to see how many vitamin A-rich foods you eat each day.

In the April 17, 1971 issue of *Science News*, three researchers at the Neurosensory Laboratory of the State University of Buffalo, New York, report that the effects of vitamin A deficiency are critically dependent on exposure to light.

Drs. W.K. Noell, M. C. Delmelle and Renate Albrecht fed rats diets in which there was not enough vitamin A. They kept them in complete darkness and found that their supply of rhodopsin (visual purple) was normal. This is the substance so rapidly destroyed by light which must be present in our eyes for good vision. Then they fed other rats a diet deficient in vitamin A and kept them on a cycle of dim light, then darkness. These animals lost their store of rhodopsin continuously.

The increase of rhodopsin in the control animals kept in complete darkness suggests, say these scientists, that light plays an important role, not only in visual deficiency but also in the normal biology of visual cells.

Astronomers have been known to complain about what they consider the most intrusive of all forms of pollution—light pollution! The light given off from large cities, from airports, from industrial plants is so bright that it often obscures their view of the night sky, making their work much more difficult. Shouldn't we all perhaps give a lot more thought to this matter of light and what it may mean to good health? Wouldn't it be wiser, perhaps, to do as the wild birds and animals do—go to bed when darkness comes and get up with the dawn, spending as little time as possible under artificial light of any kind?

We know that light falls through our eyes on the pituitary gland which is the master gland of the body. In birds and animals, this light governs most of their activities. In spring, when there is much more light, glands become very active and the mating season begins in the bird and animal world. The exact way all this comes about is not fully understood at present. But we do know the great importance of light for all the activities of birds and animals.

Why should man be an exception? Is it not possible we may discover that some of our most baffling ailments may be the result of our meddling with the cycles of darkness and light—changing night into day as it were? Isn't it possible that some of the restlessness, violence and mental illness so widespread in our urban centers may spring from the simple fact that these caged-in people simply never get enough uninterrupted time in darkness to renew whatever body elements—like the eye substance—may be destroyed by light?

Until our scientists know a great deal more about these matters, it seems the height of wisdom to assure yourself of plenty of vitamin A, especially if you work long hours under artificial light, if you stay up late, if you subject your eyes often or ever to spotlights, footlights and all that modern welter of lighting equipment which seems to give so much pleasure to so many people.

Medical World News reported on March 5, 1971 that **massive doses of vitamin A have been used in the treatment of a very serious eye disease, retinitis pigmentosa**. This condition is defined as hereditary, with slowly progressive blindness.

Two patients with clouded vision from this condition were given 200,000 units of vitamin A by a team of doctors at the National Institute of Arthritis and Metabolic Diseases in Washington, D. C. Hours after they took the vitamin, their vision began to clear. Within a day they were seeing well. The effect of this one dose of vitamin A lasted for three months! Vitamin A, remember, is stored in the body. One patient, who started treatment seven years ago now has relatively good vision. The other patient has since died of an unrelated disease (heart failure).

The eye condition, which has hitherto been considered incurable, affects children who are unable to absorb the fat-soluble vitamins. That means vitamins A, D, E and K. We wonder whether the heart failure of the one patient may have been due to simple inability to absorb vitamin E, which has often proved so useful in circulatory ailments.

Dr. Peter Goursa, who treated the patients, feels that his success may indicate that **vitamin A deficiency is at the root of most types of retinal degeneration**.

It is also interesting to note that Dr. Arthur Alexander Knapp of New York City treats retinitis pigmentosa with vitamin D and calcium supplements. He has been using this therapy for 30 years, he says in a letter to the editor of *Medical Tribune* for February 23, 1970.

What about cataracts, you may ask? Will vitamins cure this unpleasant disorder? Well, it usually doesn't happen that way. Vitamins are not drugs—even though they are sometimes used by doctors in large dosages like drugs—and you cannot cure some disease of long standing by simply taking "a vitamin" and doing nothing at all about correcting that non-nourishing diet and unhealthful way of life that had a lot to do with creating the condition in the first place. Nor is it likely to do much good to take two vitamins or three, even if you throw in a few minerals. While one vitamin may make a difference in the way you feel, after the vitamin has had some time to "work," and you may even notice some additional good effects that you had not expected, chances are that you will do much better by taking a full schedule of vitamins combined with the best possible diet and a way of life that is conducive to good health.

The fallacy of demanding that one vitamin cure one disease is highlighted by an experiment performed in the laboratory of one of the world's most distinguished biologists in the field of nutrition—Dr. Roger J. Williams of the University of Texas. All his professional life Dr. Williams has been trying to educate the general public and his professional colleagues as well as government officials to the basic principle that vitamins and minerals are not drugs—that all of them work together as a team, that there is no such thing as one vitamin or one mineral curing a disease. They must all be involved.

Says Dr. Williams in an article in the *Proceedings of the National Academy of Sciences*, October, 1974, "No nutrient by itself should be expected to prevent or cure any disease; nutrients as such always work cooperatively in metabolism as a team.... Unlike drugs, single nutrients always act constructively like parts of a complicated machine and are effective only when they participate as members of a team. This does not prevent nutrients from having drug-like actions when used in amounts higher than the physiological levels.... When particular vitamins appear to cure specific diseases, it is because they round out the team, transforming a limping incomplete team into one that is complete enough to function with some degree of physiological adequacy. ... Testing nutrients for their effectiveness is thus entirely different from testing drugs. Unless a nutrient is tested under conditions which allow it to participate in teamwork, the results are likely to be seriously misleading."

Dr. Williams and a colleague set out to test this theory on laboratory rats. It is well known that rats lack an enzyme which is necessary to use properly a sugar which appears in milk—galactose. Since they lack this enzyme, they generally get cataracts when they are fed lots of milk or milk products. The Texas researchers set up an experiment using 18 different diets. All the diets except one (the control diet) contained quite large amounts of galactose—up to 20 per cent of the diet. The rest of the diet was arranged so that some of the rats got just the usual chow which adequately nourishes laboratory rats; some diets contained nothing but eggs in addition to the galactose. An all-egg diet has been found by Dr. Williams to constitute a complete and very healthful diet for rats. Some of the diets contained the usual laboratory chow plus vitamins in quite large amounts.

At the end of nine weeks cataracts had formed in the eyes of many of the rats which got the plain chow with no vitamins. Although they were getting the same large amount of galactose (the cataract-former), those rats which got, in

41

addition, the vitamin supplements had no cataracts. In every case the number of cataracts increased in direct proportion to the lack of nutrients in the diet. Those diets which contained most in the way of vitamins, in addition to the basic good diet, produced no cataracts. Those which contained no extra vitamins did produce cataracts. The diets in between—with fewer vitamins added—produced some cataracts, but not as many as the diets with no added vitamins. The control group of rats which got no cataract-producing galactose—also had no cataracts.

In a second experiment all the rats were fed a diet designed to produce cataracts. They were then fed a good diet plus all the vitamins to see if the cataracts would regress. The results of this experiment were not as clear-cut as those of the first experiment. Of 26 cataracts, 16 showed improvement from 40 to 80 per cent. But, in general, the regressions were slow and incomplete, "though improvement in many cases was clearly manifested," says Dr. Williams. It seems that the lens of the eye (where cataracts form) has a slow rate of metabolism—that is, any improvement might be expected to be slow.

Dr. Williams points out that his experiments do not prove that one or another vitamin will prevent cataracts. Nor is it possible to decide which of the vitamins given to the test animals was responsible for preventing the cataracts. There is no way to know if leaving out one or more of the vitamins would have changed the results. There is also no way to know whether the vitamins given are in complete "balance"—that is, whether too much of one vitamin was given, perhaps, or too little of another.

The point is that, however complete the traditional nourishing laboratory diet for rats is, it can always be improved by the addition of vitamins—all the vitamins. It can be improved to such an extent that the mere addition of all these vitamins can prevent cataracts forming even when the rats are given very large amounts of a substance which is almost guaranteed to produce cataracts in rats!

How does this happen? What do the additional vitamins do to perform this near-miracle? We do not know, says Dr. Williams. It is possible that, with the extra nutrients, the animals build enzyme systems to substitute for the one they lack—the one that is necessary to handle galactose, the cataract-causing substance.

What about human beings? **Cataract is a frequent accompaniment of diabetes.** Can enough of all the vitamins provide enough extra nutritional building materials to overcome the tendency to diabetic cataracts? What about those cataracts that appear in older folks, called senile cataracts? It seems quite possible that here, too, providing the optimum nutrition—not just enough to nourish but lots more than that—may be effective in preventing these cataracts from forming.

Dr. Williams thinks, too, that by treating the cataract with "supernutrition" as he calls it, the moment it is discovered, rather than waiting until it has fully developed, we might be able to prevent it from progressing any further. And if we afflict the eye with less of the toxic substance which causes the cataract, we may be able to prevent or stop its further growth. In the case of the rats, galactose is the toxic substance. Most human beings have no problems with galactose because they have the enzyme necessary to metabolize it with no difficulty. Those few people born without this enzyme may (probably will) be afflicted with the full range of symptoms which lack of this enzyme produces— failure to thrive in infancy, jaundice, involvement of liver and spleen, mental retardation and formation of cataracts.

It seems obvious that all the many cataracts now being treated or removed from the eyes of diabetics and older folks are not the result of inability to metabolize galactose. We do not know what causes most human cataracts. **Some specialists think it may be the result of eating too much sugar, since cataract is common among us Westerners who consume such large amounts of sugar.** No matter what it is that causes human cataracts, doesn't it seem possible that they might be prevented by following the design of the experiment described above?

Eat the most highly nourishing diet possible, like the laboratory chow which nourished the rats. Then add vitamins to achieve supernutrition. The best way to achieve the most nourishing diet for human beings is to eliminate sugar from your meals and snacks. Many modern people eat so much sugar and refined white flour products that half of the meals consist of these two foods. There is little that nourishes in either of these foods except for starch, sugar and otherwise empty calories. Laboratory rats die of malnutrition when they are fed diets like this.

Once you have eliminated the twin hazards of refined sugar and refined cereal and bread products, everything else that you eat is nourishing. There's no need to plan outlandish, difficult or expensive meals. Just be sure that you include the high protein foods, plus all the seed foods like wholegrains, bran, wheat germ, seeds of all kinds, nuts, soybeans, peas, beans, peanuts, all the fruits and vegetables, especially those that have lots of bright yellow and/or green. Eating this kind of diet—as widely varied as possible—you will get the same highly nourishing food as the laboratory rats had.

Then, according to Dr. Williams' experiments, add to that excellent diet all the known vitamins, some of them in quite large amounts. The chart on Page 49 shows the amounts of vitamins Dr. Williams used for his animals. No vitamin C is included, since rats make their own vitamin C and do not need to get it in food. You, however, need it very decidedly and you should add comparatively large amounts of it to your supplement program.

To calculate the amounts for human diets, estimate the number of calories you eat each day. It's probably in the neighborhood of about 3,000 for an adult man and about 2,000 for an adult woman. These are the official recommended number of calories for people who are of average weight and height. The nutrients given in the chart are for every 100 calories of food. If you are eating 3,000 calories multiply the numbers in the chart by 30 to get an estimate of how much you should be taking to achieve what was achieved in the rat experiment.

While on the subject of eyes, **vitamin B2 (riboflavin) has been mentioned often in relation to eye health**. Adelle Davis in *Let's Get Well* says that lack of riboflavin may produce these symptoms: sensitivity to bright light, inability to see well in dim light, watery eyes, bloodshot or painful eyes, itching or "sandy" eyelids, blurred or dim vision, eyestrain after close work, conjunctivitis, iritis, rubiosis iritis, flickering or disappearing images before the eyes, halos around bright lights or objects, dark spots before the eyes, corneal opacities. These are also symptoms of other conditions that may not be caused by lack of riboflavin. Cataracts have been produced in animals by withholding riboflavin. See that you get enough of it. It's not easy if you avoid dairy products and liver, which are the richest sources. Nuts, brewers yeast and dark green leafy vegetables are also good sources.

Vitamin C appears to be almost a specific for good eye health. In his fine book, *The Healing Factor, Vitamin C Against Disease*, Dr. Irwin Stone tells us that, in 1962, a biochemist found 12 separate biochemical processes that go on inside your eye which involve vitamin C. It has been known since 1930, says Stone, that vitamin C is found in the eye at much higher levels than in the blood or in many other body tissues. Eyes of animals, for example, contain the vitamin in these amounts: the cornea, 30 milligrams; the lens (that part of the eye which is affected by cataract) 34 milligrams; the retina 22; compared to only 2 milligrams in muscles, 4 in heart, 13 in kidney and 17 in brain. Adrenal glands, which protect us from stress, may contain as much as 160 milligrams of vitamin C, the pituitary gland 126.

Dr. Stone believes that **vitamin C may be protective against glaucoma**, the disorder involving high pressure within the eyeball which presses on the optic nerve and eventually destroys sight. In 1964, a Swedish doctor gave 500 milligrams of vitamin C twice daily and produced a significant drop in eyeball pressure. He later treated glaucoma patients with 2 grams (2,000 milligrams) of vitamin C daily and got decreases in pressure.

From 1965 to 1969, many papers published in the scientific and medical journals of other nations reported on reduction of pressure in the eye using vitamin C. One such paper reported the use of intravenous injections of sodium ascorbate (one form of vitamin C) at doses of about 70 grams per day, with no side effects. Pressure in the eyes was promptly reduced. Dr. Stone points out that no work along these lines has apparently been done in our country, although "numerous government bulletins have appeared describing the urgent need for solving the problem of glaucoma." He asks for immediate research on the possibility of preventing glaucoma by taking three to five grams of vitamin C daily. And using it in higher doses both orally and intravenously for glaucoma that has already developed.

Dr. Stone tells us that there is a marked decrease in certain kinds of chemical substances in the eye with cataract. Scientists have questioned whether possibly the high levels of vitamin C found in eyes are there to protect against the loss of these essential elements by oxidation. **In parts of the world where cataracts are extremely common even in very young people there is a much lower concentration of vitamin C in these diseased eyes.**

As long ago as 1941, British physicians reported dramatic improvement in eyes which had been injured by disease and accidents when vitamin C was given intravenously in very large doses, even though the patients showed no signs of vitamin C deficiency. In 1939, two Argentinian physicians obtained good results in 90 per cent of 60 patients with daily injections of vitamin C (50 to 100 milligrams). A Detroit physician gave 350 milligrams daily and got improvement in 60 per cent of his patients. Such therapeutic doses are considered small in comparison with the massive doses being given today successfully for various complaints.

Dr. Donald T. Atkinson, an ophthalmologist with more than 30 years experience, gave one gram (1,000 milligrams) of vitamin C daily to 450 patients with "incipient cataract."

Although Dr. Stone does not mention it, Dr. Atkinson also put his patients who were about to have problems with cataracts on excellent highly nourishing diets, including two eggs and a pint of milk every day, plus lots of dark green leafy vegetables fresh from the garden if possible, and all the fresh raw fruit they could eat. And he gave them 200,000 units of vitamin A daily. One should not take this much vitamin A except under a doctor's supervision, for some people have had unpleasant side effects, since the vitamin is stored in the body and accumulates. But certainly taking up to 25,000 units of vitamin A daily is quite harmless and very beneficial.

Over a period of 11 years, the cataracts remained "incipient" in many of these patients and needed no further treatment or surgery. Dr. Stone says there is also evidence that large amounts of vitamin C may be helpful in preventing retinal detachment, another prevalent eye disorder.

In *New Hope for Incurable Diseases*, Drs. E. Cheraskin and W. M. Ringsdorf, Jr. devote one chapter to **glaucoma**. Approximately two million Americans suffer from this dreaded disease. No two cases are alike so one cannot generalize. These two medical researchers recommend giving up coffee and tea, or severely limiting them, as well as excessive smoking. Don't spend long hours every week in darkness with your eyes open—at the movies, for example. Don't use sunglasses excessively.

They also mention a paper given by four Italian physicians at a meeting in Rome. These doctors had given as much as 35 grams of vitamin C daily to a group of glaucoma patients and had achieved a highly significant drop in intraocular pressure. The drop in pressure reached its lowest point about four to five hours after the vitamin dose was taken. It was maintained for more than eight hours. Most patients given this much vitamin C in a single dose developed diarrhea. So the dose was divided into five doses during the day. The patients had no more trouble with diarrhea and, for periods of 45 days, it was possible to obtain acceptable pressure in the eyes of many patients, even those whose pressure could not be controlled with oral drugs or eye drops.

A British scientist reported in 1959 that children who are very short-sighted (myopic) can improve if given high protein diets. In children over 12, the greatest improvement occurred always in those children who were getting the most protein. And a French doctor gave 100 milligram tablets of vitamin E in divided doses during the day to a group of children and got improvement in their myopia. There's no harm in trying it with your own children if they must wear glasses because of myopia.

One of the most common vision problems among Americans may be partially the result of a low-protein, high-carbohydrate diet, according to Dr. Theodore Grosvenor. Writing in the *Journal of the American Optometric Association*, July, 1976, Dr. Grosvenor of Indiana University's School of Optometry says the condition known as **astigmatism** has long been thought to be due to pressure of the eyelids against the eye. A low-protein, high-carbohydrate diet may result in a lowering of ocular rigidity to the point that even normal pressure from the eyelids would cause astigmatism, he says.

Astigmatism refers to an irregularity in the shape of the front surface or cornea of the eye. A recent review of records in California, revealed that from 75 to 80 per cent of the prescriptions written through the California Vision Services contained a correction for astigmatism.

Higher degrees of astigmatism cause distorted or blurred vision, according to the American Optometric Association. Smaller degrees usually cause symptoms of eyestrain—headache, fatigue, loss of achievement, etc.

Studies of astigmatism among different age groups, ethnic groups and contact lens wearers has led Dr. Grosvenor to conclude that astigmatism may also be caused by pressure from the eyelids to contact lenses on eyes that are too soft.

Although the human eye is not completely hard, it does have a degree of rigidity maintained by the fluid inside the eye. In the normal eye, there is sufficient rigidity to maintain a smooth round outer surface of the eye. It is possible that this rigidity could be reduced by improper diet, the Association says.

Dr. Grosvenor also reports that the wearing of contact lenses sometimes induces astigmatism and that the degree of the condition decreases with age. He attributes the latter to a loss of eyelid pressure that comes with the aging process.

Getting back to cataracts and vitamin C, three scientists at the Laboratory of Vision Research, National Eye Institute at Bethesda, Maryland think they have found a substance or substances which may help to prevent cataracts. The

---

Nutrients (Per 100 Calories) Furnished by Vitamin Mixture in Diets Which Prevented Cataracts

Vitamin A	1,333 I.U.
Vitamin D3	66.7 I.U.
Vitamin E	40 milligrams
Thiamine	0.83 milligrams
Riboflavin	1.67 milligrams
Niacin	10 milligrams
Pantothenic acid	5.3 milligrams
Pyridoxine	0.8 milligrams
Vitamin B12	3.3 micrograms
Folic acid	3.3 milligrams
Biotin	70 micrograms
Choline	50 milligrams
Inositol	33.3 milligrams

Plus some vitamin K and some fatty acid mixes.

---

substances are flavonoids which were once studied with great care as potentially very valuable substances that exist mostly in fruits and vegetables in association with vitamin C. They consist of a number of related substances called by various names: hesperidin, citrin, rutin and so on. Your health food store carries them, usually under the name of bioflavonoids, or else as rutin or hesperidin. They are often included in vitamin C supplements as they apparently help vitamin C perform its various biological functions.

The Eye Institute scientists used various flavonoids in conjunction with the lenses of eyes taken from animals. They put the two together in test tubes and found that the flavonoids prevented the appearance of the enzyme which causes the cataract to form on the lens of the eye. This is an enzyme called *aldose reductase*, which reacts with galactose, the sugar found in milk, and begins the formation of the cataract. In other words, so far as test tube work is concerned, you need only add a given amount of one or several flavonoids and no cataract material will be formed in the lens.

Several of the flavonoids were more effective than others in preventing the appearance of the undesirable cataract-forming enzyme. But it seems possible that by using more of the less effective ones, the same effect might be achieved.

Say the authors of this article, which appeared in *Science* for June 20, 1975, "Since flavonoids are relatively nontoxic, the present finding that some of them are the most potent inhibitors of *aldose reductase* known so far suggests that they may be useful in preventing the onset of diabetic or galactosemic cataracts...."

A number of years ago researchers were doing a lot of work on bioflavonoids. These natural substances were found to help in preventing colds. They were found to be effective in preventing the breakage of small capillaries. They were found to be useful in treating various ear conditions where hardening of the arteries was probably involved.

Then the Food and Drug Administration stepped in and announced that makers of health foods and food supplements were forbidden to advertise bioflavonoids as essential to health or as contributing anything to health, in spite of all the laboratory evidence indicating their usefulness in many conditions.

But many people still wanted the bioflavonoids and found that they improved their health in many ways. So they are still being sold in health food stores. Now it appears that they may have a value which was unknown until recently. They can and do destroy the enzyme which manufactures the cataract-causing substance in some kinds of cataracts.

We have no evidence yet as to how or when they may be used by physicians to prevent cataract or restrain its growth. Nor do we have any idea whether they will ever be available in any form that might be distilled into the eye where the cataract is forming.

But this is no reason we cannot make use of bioflavonoid preparations and eat lots of the fruits in which they appear. This is one good reason to eat the white segments of citrus fruits. The bioflavonoids are concentrated there. So don't always juice your oranges or grapefruit. Eat them, including the white segments. And when you make homemade orange or grapefruit juice, leave all pulp in the juice and drink it.

Generally speaking, bioflavonoids occur most abundantly in those foods which contain the most vitamin C: the citrus fruits, strawberries, green peppers, acerola cherries, rose hips and so on. Get plenty of them in food or take them in supplements. And guard against cataracts in other ways as well: by eating the most nutritious diet possible and attaining "supernutrition," if you can, by supplementing it with plenty of vitamins and minerals.

CHAPTER 5

Vitamin A and Skin Conditions

DR. IRWIN I. LUBOWE of New York is a dermatologist who uses vitamin preparations in treating various skin diseases. We are deeply obliged to him for a paper he delivered in 1974, which was reprinted in the Spring, 1975 *Journal of Applied Nutrition*. Dr. Lubowe believes that vitamin therapy can be used successfully in a number of puzzling and difficult skin conditions.

We know that vitamin A has, as one of its functions, the protection and health of the linings of body organs and the skin. Lack of vitamin A produces "horny" patches on the skin—hard, scaly patches. For some time, Dr. Lubowe tells us, dermatologists have been trying vitamin A for acne treatment. Some have found that taking rather large doses of vitamin A—but not large enough to be toxic—affects the skin in such a way that the primary lesion of acne—the pimple—is not formed.

One dermatologist says that vitamin A can be absorbed through the skin. He finds **the following conditions are related to vitamin A deficiency:** dry, weak and brittle hair, acne, *ichthyosis* (dry, harsh scaly skin), *keratosis follicularia* (warty, crusted patches on skin), *leukoplakia* (a thick, white area), which is frequently pre-cancerous, *seborrhea* (oily coating in the form of scales or crusts), *folliculitis* (inflammation of a hair follicle), *keratosis palmaris* and a number of other skin conditions, as well as (in some cases) white spots and ridges on fingernails.

Now a form of vitamin A called retinoic acid is being used by dermatologists to treat **acne**. This treatment takes a long time—up to six weeks—and produces an unsightly skin during the process. Dr. Lubowe tells us that many dermatologists regularly prescribe 25,000 to 50,000 units of vitamin A daily to prevent acne.

The January, 1974 *Dermatology News* reported beneficial use of retinoic acid (a form of vitamin A) for treating **leukoplakia**, which, as we stated, is a thick, white area on the mucus membrane and keratotic or horny skin patches. These doctors applied a 0.1 per cent solution of the vitamin A product from one to three times daily. Treatment was given from three to 14 days, interrupted by seven to 15 days to prevent irritation, then repeated.

Among the B vitamins, **riboflavin is known as another protector of the health of the skin**. Lack of riboflavin brings seborrhea, that oily skin disease which produces scales and crusts at various parts of the body. Mouth, tongue and the corners of the mouth are also affected in riboflavin deficiency, as well as inflammation of the eyelids. There is also discomfort in bright light.

In **pellagra**, the disease of niacin (vitamin B3) deficiency, the skin becomes crusted and scarred, especially on parts of the body where sunlight falls—hands and face chiefly. Ample amounts of niacin, along with a good high-protein diet, eliminate such dermatitis very quickly. Forty years ago nutrition experts were giving brewers yeast to pellagra victims—whole cups of it every day, because of its niacin content. It brought about a speedy cure of this serious, often fatal disease.

A deficiency in vitamin B6 (pyridoxine) can bring about **seborrhea** of the face and scalp, says Dr. Lubowe, as well as inflammation of the tongue. Pyridoxine has also been mentioned in connection with many other disorders of skin, digestion and nerves. It is often used in massive doses by those psychiatrists who treat schizophrenia with large doses of vitamins. It is water soluble, so any excess not used by the body is excreted daily. You need have no fear of getting too much of this important B vitamin.

Vitamin B12 is usually thought of in connection with preventing pernicious anemia. It occurs only in foods of animal origin like meat, poultry, eggs, fish and milk, so completely vegetarian diets are likely to be almost completely devoid of this essential nutrient. Dermatologists have reported seborrhea occurring as a result of disturbed carbohydrate metabolism plus lack of vitamin B12. Injections of the vitamin produced remission. Very often in such patients it is important to inject the vitamin, rather than giving it by mouth, since the victim may not be able to absorb vitamin B12 from the digestive tract.

There have been reports of a peculiar pigmentation which accompanies pernicious anemia and which vitamin B12 injections cure. One physician has reported that he coaxed some pigment back into the hair and skin of a patient by giving large doses of pyridoxine every day for three years. When the vitamin was withheld, the pigment began to fade once more.

Dr. Lubowe prescribes bioflavonoids along with vitamin C to disperse dilated capillaries on the cheeks and nose. He gives 400 to 800 milligrams of these for a long time, he says. The Food and Drug Administration has steadfastly claimed that bioflavonoids have no place in human nutrition and are not essential food elements. But again and again innovative physicians have used them, usually in conjunction with vitamin C, to achieve good health. They occur along with vitamin C in fruits, berries and vegetables.

The list of skin disorders which respond well to vitamin E is a long one. We will briefly discuss some of these. Dr. Lubowe quotes Dr. Samuel Ayers, Jr. of Los Angeles, who has used the vitamin in the following disorders. **The doses used are very large—up to 2,000 International Units per day.**

Epidermolysis bullosa, a painful, disfiguring disease in which the skin is covered with blisters.

Granuloma annulare—purple or reddish patches usually on arms or legs.

Scleroderma—an accumulation of collagen in the skin.

Lichen sclerosus—white patches on skin with hair follicles plugged with keratin. Usually affects the neck, the trunk, the vulva and the penis.

Necrobiosis lipidica—yellow to red plaques on arms or legs. This usually occurs in diabetics.

Lupus erythematosus—the dermatitis is only one aspect of this generalized disorder.

Restless legs or cramps—pins and needles or cramps in legs and feet.

Raynaud's phenomenon—pallor or bluish color in fingers or toes caused by poor circulation.

Swiss physicians treated 24 patients with **psoriasis** using retinoic acid in the form of RO 10-9359. This is a compound derived from vitamin A. The amounts of the compound that were given must have been very large, since the account, in a Swiss medical journal, states that the effects of getting "too much" vitamin A were "slight to marked." Only in patients with very severe psoriasis was the effectiveness of the medication deemed to be worth the side effects.

It is not the purpose of this book, or any of our books, to deal in cures or treatments. But if vitamin A preparations are indeed effective in treating a number of skin conditions, does it not seem possible that getting plenty of vitamin A in foods and food supplements throughout one's lifetime will help to avoid these pesky skin disorders?

The disfiguring skin condition called **ichthyosis** is yielding to a vitamin A preparation applied to the skin, according to *Medical World News.* The preparation, as noted above, is retinoic acid.

Two Wisconsin children, aged 11 and 12, suffered from this condition in which the skin looks like fish scales. Some forms of the disease are hereditary. They had been treated with antibiotics on the skin and taken internally, compresses, emolients to soften the skin, kerolytics (drugs which cause the outer layers of the skin to slough off), and vitamin A by mouth. Nothing had ever improved their condition. Their father also suffered from the condition and no treatments had helped him either.

Dr. William F. Schorr of the Marshfield Clinic, Marshfield, Wisconsin, has been treating the girls unsuccessfully since their birth. Finally, he tried retinoic acid. In this case, the preparation is made by Johnson and Johnson under the trade name of Retin-A.

The younger girl applied the ointment to half of her abdomen in order that any improvement in the condition could be compared to the other untreated half. Within three weeks the thick, horny, foul-smelling crust on the treated skin was clear. Nothing remained but a mild redness. Both children were hospitalized for a thorough test. The ointment was applied two to three times daily and both children improved almost at once. The father was given ointment to apply all over his body and there was considerable improvement.

Doctors and patients alike could easily see improvement. But when the doctors examined the skin under the microscope the great change was apparent. Normal skin has overlapping cells so that there is continuous protection to the layers of skin underneath. But in the "alligator" kind of skin, which this disease produces, there are masses of heaped up cells separated by deep crevices. In these crevices bacteria lodge. Since no amount of washing will remove them, they produce foul odors which are one of the distressing aspects of the disease.

Skin specimens taken after treatment with Retin-A showed that the deep crevices had disappeared, the skin cells were growing much more naturally and overlapping one another as they should. And the number of bacteria on the skin were considerably reduced. Dr. Schorr stated that the drug is "more than just a salve to produce skin scaling. The normalization of the entire skin parallels the remarkable clinical improvement."

Dr. James E. Fulton of the Department of Dermatology at the University of Miami School of Medicine, agrees. He has treated several patients with this form of vitamin A, which he calls, "probably the only useful treatment we now have for ichthyosis."

And Dr. Phillip Frost, co-chief of the skin and cancer unit of the Mt. Sinai Medical Center of Greater Miami has treated about 40 victims of this disease and has found the **vitamin A preparation successful in the severe forms of the disease**. It seems that it may be necessary for these people to use this preparation for the rest of their lives, but this is surely a small price to pay for relief from such a disfiguring and disagreeable condition.

All the doctors who are using the salve treat it as a drug and are concerned apparently only with curing their patients. But doesn't it seem very possible that such a condition, from birth, must be caused by some gross malfunction of all the body mechanisms that process vitamin A? Perhaps treatment of the mother and father with large doses of vitamin A before the children are conceived might prevent this condition.

Getting back to **psoriasis**, 22 patients were treated with retinoic acid and found significant improvement, according to the *New York State Journal of Medicine*, Volume 11, January, 1973, pages 2584-2587. They were also given cortisone at the same time. We are not told what part this may have played in the improvement. In the same journal, we learn of a case of severe liver damage caused by treatment of psoriasis by a more familiar drug—methotrexate—which is given for psoriasis.

One reason why many people may be having trouble with disorders which vitamin A may treat is explained in *The*

Lancet for November 24, 1973. Five physicians from the University of Chicago describe 13 patients who had no symptoms of vitamin deficiency but who were suffering from chronic conditions of the small intestine.

All these patients were studied carefully to see if there were any signs of vitamin A deficiency. There were none except for one patient who said she had trouble driving at night. She could not see well enough. The conditions which had brought these patients to the hospital were: jejunal diverticulosis, regional enteritis and celiac sprue. In all of these it is suspected that considerable amounts of vitamins as well as fats and proteins may not be absorbed well. But there appeared to be no deficiencies among these patients.

Ten of the patients had been taking vitamin supplements which contained from 3,500 to 10,000 units of vitamin A. Nevertheless, the Chicago doctors decided to test them all with a "dark adaptation" test which is a certain test for vitamin A deficiency. They all failed it. In other words, all these patients were trying to get along on far less vitamin A than they needed just for good vision, especially good vision after dark.

The entire group was given 50,000 units of vitamin A daily for one month and only two failed to improve in their "dark adaptation" test. These were two elderly women with celiac sprue.

The doctors speculate on what may have caused the deficiency without any other symptoms. Well, perhaps these people just don't store vitamin A in their bodies as they should, due to the problem they have with not absorbing food. It's also possible, the physicians believe, that they may also be suffering from other vitamin deficiencies which were never discovered. Disturbances of the retina (that part of the eye which is involved in night-time vision) also occur when people are not getting enough thiamine or riboflavin—two B vitamins.

Deficiencies in riboflavin and vitamin C may produce delayed dark adaptation—that is, the eye requires a long time before it can see in darkness or near darkness. But vitamin A is the chief vitamin involved probably, although in people who do not absorb one vitamin chances are they will not absorb other nutrients either. And as their nutritional deficiencies worsen, they will probably absorb still less of these essential elements, producing a vicious cycle.

Say the Chicago doctors, "The high frequency of subclinical vitamin A deficiency found in this group suggests that occult (hidden) nutritional deficiency may be more prevalent in patients with intestinal disease than is commonly appreciated. Routine vitamin supplementation cannot be relied upon to prevent the functional deficit demonstrated in this study."

We do not know how many people in this country suffer from these conditions. We doubt that anyone knows, for many such sufferers probably do not even go to doctors. What we do know is that such invalids need far more vitamin A than they can normally get in their diet. **For that reason, vitamin A supplements are certainly recommended.**

"**Acne** is constantly present in epidemic proportions. At any given time 60 per cent to 90 per cent of teenagers are afflicted." This quote from a physician appeared in the May, 1959 *Medical Clinics of North America.* A University of Pennsylvania skin specialist, speaking at a 1974 symposium on dermatology said that acne now afflicts 100 per cent of the population. Every young person has acne, Dr. Albert Kligman stated, and it is incorrect to speak of those with and without acne, although the disease may range from very mild to very acute forms.

One might assume from these two statistics that in the short space of 13 years as much as 40 per cent of the youthful population acquired this disease. And so it seems. Very few doctors question why this should be. How does it happen that an unsightly, embarrassing and annoying skin condition which is unknown among primitive people and was almost unknown among Westerners 50 years ago should, today, afflict 100 per cent of adolescents in our country, if Dr. Kligman's figures are correct?

Dr. Kligman is one of three University of Pennsylvania skin specialists who treat acne with retinoic acid. In serious cases where the acne "pimples" are badly infected, they give antibiotics as well. And in some cases they give massive, potentially toxic doses of vitamin A for brief periods of time.

Could one say, then, that acne is caused by lack of vitamins? It seems unlikely, for these doctors are using the vitamin A acid preparation as a salve in highly concentrated form. It produces some startling effects which seems to have no relation to the usual activities of vitamin A in body cells. But, they tell us, they have found no toxicity, no harmful effects from the use of retinoic acid.

In a major article in *Postgraduate Medicine*, February, 1974, Dr. Kligman and his colleagues, Otto H. Mills and James J. Leyden, tell us that "Acne is a serious disease in a society whose consciousness of cosmetic comeliness has been raised to narcissistic obsession." In past years treatment of the disease involved all kinds of things, none of them successful, and millions of young people attained adulthood permanently scarred with the leavings of acne "pimples" or comedones, as doctors call them.

The acne pimple forms in a skin follicle having glands in which sebum is secreted. This is an oily substance. And acne victims have oily skin. As the horny mass grows larger, a tiny whitehead of pus appears, to be followed by a horny mass crowned by a "blackhead." As these pustules break or are pressed out, infected material is carried to adjoining cells. The skin, trying to heal the wound, may enclose the whole thing in a layer of skin, resulting in a festering, draining nodule which just doesn't heal. "This is the worst manifestation," say the three skin specialists, "invariably resulting in scarring."

At the University of Pennsylvania, **acne is treated with vitamin A acid salve—"a potent agent."** Applied very tenderly to the skin and not rubbed in, it produces redness and peeling. And, at first for a month or two, it produces more comedones than before. The acne has apparently grown worse. But after about 10 weeks the redness and peeling disappear and the manifestations of acne gradually disappear as well.

The doctors do not promise quick success. The value of the vitamin A salve can be estimated after about eight weeks, they tell us, and with greater certainty at 12 weeks. The patient should continue to use the salve for as long as there appears to be the chance of more pimples appearing. If it is stopped before that time, there will be a relapse. So it should not be stopped until signs of the disease have completely disappeared. However, "among hundreds of patients who have used tretinoin (the vitamin A acid preparation) daily for as long as two to three years, we have not encountered serious or irreversible local side effects. Systemic effects are unknown," say the Pennsylvania specialists.

If inflammation is severe, antibiotics should also be prescribed as well. They should be withdrawn as soon as the disease is "stabilized." And vitamin A can be given orally at the same time. They give vitamin A in a dosage of 100,000 International Units a day for one week. Then they raise it gradually to 400,000 units daily for a short time, then gradually reduce the dosage, then withdraw it entirely. There are unpleasant symptoms: headache, nausea, itching, dry skin may be noticed. After all, it is well known that vitamin A is toxic in these extremely large amounts, so no one should ever dose himself in such a manner for long periods of time.

So much for treating acne. And, as is often the case, these doctors who are getting such fine results see no hope for preventing the disease—by changing the diet, for instance. Diet has absolutely nothing to do with it, they say. And to forbid teenagers their favorite foods—candy, chocolate, soft drinks, fried foods, ice cream—is just too cruel, they continue, since none of these has anything to do with causing acne.

We cannot help but wonder why no surprise is expressed

61

by these physicians at the fact that acne is a relatively new disease, unknown to our ancestors. And that it is also unknown among primitive people everywhere who may suffer from many kinds of skin disorders caused by the harsh conditions in which they live, lack of hygiene and soap, infections caused by parasites and insects, and so on. But not acne. They do not suffer from acne.

In the case of the Eskimos, acne appears readily as soon as these primitive people move to town where "store" food is easily and inexpensively available. They become "sugar addicts," consuming vast amounts of soft drinks, chocolates, bakery products, candy, etc. And pimples appear almost overnight in the young people.

Primitive Eskimos lived almost entirely on protein and fat (meat and fish containing large amounts of fat). As their traditional foods have disappeared, due to the encroachment of "civilization," they move to town and begin to live on the easily available, generally inexpensive, high-carbohydrate, high-sugar diet they can buy at the store.

Results in terms of health are catastrophic, according to every medical observer. Dr. Otto Schaefer in *Nutrition Today*, November/December, 1971 tells us their children grow faster and taller, their teeth rot, women rapidly succumb to gall bladder diseases; they become fat, they are beginning to succumb to diabetes and hardening of the arteries, heart attacks—and acne.

"We have reason to believe," says Dr. Schaefer, "that the great and rapid increase in consumption of sucrose (sugar) especially if taken, as is increasingly the case, without preceding meat meals—may have serious metabolic-endocrine repercussions." He means glandular effects which disrupt blood sugar levels and digestion.

Acne is completely unknown among Eskimos eating their traditional diet which includes no refined and processed carbohydrates.

"Today," says Dr. Schaefer, "many Eskimos themselves blame their pimples on the 'pop-chocolate and candies' their children consume as if addicted. One wonders what these people and other old Northerners would think if they were told to read some recent medical publications, in which dermatologists belittle or deny the role of dietary factors in the pathogenesis (cause) of acne vulgaris."

Town-dwelling Eskimos are at present eating 200 pounds of sugar per person every year. And acne has rapidly followed, as surely as night follows day. It seems reasonable, does it not, that today's children in American cities, afflicted as they almost universally are, with acne, are certainly headed for adulthood and middle-age burdened with those other afflictions of sugar-addicts—diabetes, gall bladder disorders, heart and circulatory disorders, hardening of the arteries?

"The people I studied in some of the rural areas of Ireland had little acne and virtually no visible scar tissue," said Dr. Richard Boggs, medical sociology professor of Ball State University. But people around Muncie, Indiana have, he said, more serious problems with acne than any place he ever visited.

He stated, in a UPI report, November 28, 1974, that Irish youngsters don't snack or throng to hamburger stands, as American young people do. "They definitely do not eat as many items that have been deep-fat fried," he continued. "I can say that the Irish are a fasting people whose food habits are not affected by the gluttony of affluence."

He thinks, he said, that hamburgers, french fries and soft drinks may be a major factor in the skin disease which afflicts almost all American teenagers.

"What is surprising about Irish youth," said Dr. Boggs, "is the uniform high quality of complexions in Ireland, not just the absence of acne lesions. The coloration is fantastic. Those young people are almost all rosy-cheeked. It suggests that a very healthful lifestyle contributes to one's general appearance and also is the first defense against acne."

He agrees that it is difficult to pinpoint all factors that may contribute to acne. He thinks that other aspects of life aside from dietary ones may be social stress, lack of exercise and a different climate or weather pattern.

If you or someone in your family has acne, what's the best course to take? Can you buy retinoic acid at the drug store? No. It must be administered by a doctor. Should you take massive doses of vitamin A in an effort to treat the acne? Under no circumstances. It has produced very serious side effects in people who tried this. Should you ask your doctor for antibiotics to control the skin infections? Your doctor can be the judge of this. Should you take cortisone or use cortisone skin preparations to control the acne? The Pennsylvania specialists say, "Never, never apply corticosteroid to the face of an adolescent for more than a few weeks, regardless of diagnosis." It may eventually produce permanent scarring of the face.

First of all, seek out a doctor who will treat you with retinoic acid. If your family doctor does not know of this treatment, ask him to get in touch with the Pennsylvania specialists. Once you begin the retinoic acid treatment, stop all other local treatments. Do not wash excessively with soap of any kind. Wash only once a day. Do not apply the vitamin A salve just after you have washed your face. Dry skin thoroughly first. Do not get sunburned. The vitamin A acid increases your susceptibility to sunburn. Guard against it. Wear a hat, scarf, sleeves when you are in the hot sunlight. Or stay in the shade.

Finally, why not try the primitive diet of the Eskimos to see whether you can stop the disorder in its tracks? Eat nothing but high protein foods. No carbohydrate. None at all. Or as little as possible. Eat meat, poultry, fish, shellfish, eggs, milk and cheese. As you gradually discover how much better you feel on such a diet, how much less tired you get, how your craving for sweets gradually disappears, you can begin to add those foods which are high in protein but also contain a goodly amount of unprocessed carbohydrate: seeds and nuts, peanuts, soybeans, wheat germ and bran, wholegrain breads and cereals. And, of course, salads and other vegetables. Then fruits which have the least carbohydrate.

For such a program you will, of course, continue taking your food supplements, for some vitamins are lacking in the high protein diet—vitamin C for instance. So take your vitamins every day.

And shun like the skin poisons they are foods like these: soft drinks, candy, chocolate, sugar in any form, bakery products, doughnuts, any kind of pasta and any other food which consists mostly of white sugar and/or white flour. Good luck to you!

Some time ago an article in *Obstetrics and Gynecology News* reported that teenage girls bothered with premenstrual acne found that taking pyridoxine (vitamin B6) before and during menstruation reduced their problems with this condition. And we have heard reports that a number of health seekers have completely cured their acne with lactobacillus tablets from their health food store. Take the tablets two or three times a day if you have a bad case, we are told. Once the unsightly pimples are controlled, take one tablet a day from then on.

Admittedly the report about the acidophilus capsules is not very scientific, but it did work for one 26-year-old woman so why not try it if you have a stubborn case of acne? Acne may be caused by the wrong kind of intestinal bacteria, so the acidophilus culture is beneficial in correcting this condition.

It makes sense to us. What we eat determines to a large extent the kind of intestinal bacteria we have. A diet high in fiber (wholegrains, bran, fruit and vegetables, nuts, seeds) produces one kind of intestinal bacteria. A diet in which refined carbohydrates predominate (sugar and white flour) has little fiber and produces a different kind of bacteria. The acidophilus bacteria present in yogurt (if it hasn't been destroyed by heating and pasteurization), buttermilk and tablets available at health food stores maintain good health in the intestine.

Of course, vitamins and other food supplements are not panaceas for ills caused by bad diet in general. The condition of your skin and hair is symptomatic of the condition of your general health. As your health improves with the best possible diet—and not a single mouthful wasted on empty calorie goodies—the health of your skin and hair will improve progressively—not overnight but in due time.

CHAPTER 6

Vitamin A for Cancer Prevention

MANY RECENT EXPERIMENTS have shown a direct relationship between getting enough vitamin A and cancer prevention. Those are not just educated guesses. Laboratory scientists set up elaborate experiments in which they exposed groups of mice or rats to known cancer-causing chemicals or pollutants. They gave one group of animals quite large amounts of vitamin A before the experiment started. The other group got just their regular chow. **In every experiment, the animals which had the vitamin A fortification of their diets did not get the expected cancer. Those without it did.**

According to Michael B. Sporn, M.D., of the National Cancer Institute, writing in *Nutrition Reviews* for April, 1977, such experiments have been conducted in regard to cancer of the trachea (windpipe), the bronchus (those branches of the windpipe that enter the lungs), the uterine cervix, the stomach and the vagina.

"The data at hand clearly indicate that no human population at risk for development of cancer should be allowed to remain in a vitamin A-deficient state," Dr. Sporn said. "Considering the relatively trivial cost of supplementation of the diet with a minimum daily requirement of (vitamin A) this is certainly a goal which should be met for the entire population."

The explanation given by biologists goes like this. **Vitamin A is directly responsible for controlling the way cells divide in the epithelial tissues of the body.** These are the tissues of the skin, and the linings of all body openings, like the mouth, the digestive tract, the reproductive organs and the breathing apparatus. Cells divide normally so long as enough vitamin A is present. And they develop into just the appropriate kind of cell for that part of the body.

For example, where the body operation of that part requires the use of cilia (those tiny hair-like projections that have many helpful functions), vitamin A sees to it that this kind of cell is produced. Where there is a need for mucus as in parts of the respiratory tract, **vitamin A is the most important nutritional element needed to produce just this kind of cell**. Tissues lining the bladder and uterus need another kind of cell. It can't be manufactured unless enough vitamin A is present.

Cancer is, to put it simply, a disruption of the process of cell division and differentiation. In the body that has cancer, certain cells do not reproduce themselves normally. They produce cancerous cells instead. And, in many kinds of cancer, they produce these cells rapidly and profusely, so that the body is overwhelmed with these sick cells which obstruct healthy organs and tissues, eventually causing death.

Drugs, surgery and radiation cannot, of course, change the way cells are reproducing. All they do is to destroy the sick cells in the hope of eliminating the cancer from the body. But getting enough vitamin A will apparently prevent the entire disease process from getting started—at least in those parts of the body where epithelial cells are present, as listed above.

Well and good, one would think. All we need to do is to get enough vitamin A every day and we're forever safe from fear of getting cancer. But it's not quite that simple. First, the exposure to chemical cancer causers (or carcinogens) may be so overwhelming (as in the case of workers exposed to carcinogens at their work or chain smokers exposed continuously to the many carcinogens in cigarette smoke) that one simply cannot get enough vitamin A to give complete protection. **Then, too, you may be one of those people who need far more vitamin A than someone else,** even in your family, so that exposure to carcinogens would increase your requirements so greatly there would be no way to get enough of this vitamin.

And this leads us to the final problem, which Dr. Sporn takes up in his *Reviews* article. Natural vitamin A, supplements of which come mostly from fish liver oils, is toxic if you get too much of it. The reason is that whatever you don't need on a daily basis is stored in your liver. And taking very large doses over a long period of time overwhelms your liver and may cause unpleasant and sometimes dangerous complications. Then, too, Dr. Sporn tells us, much of the natural vitamin A may not be able to reach tissues in such organs as the bladder because of the way this vitamin is transported in the blood.

These are the reasons why laboratory scientists have developed synthetic forms of vitamin A with a molecule changed here and there, so that they are not stored in the liver and can be given in immense doses to their experimental animals. These compounds cannot do some of the other things natural vitamin A does. Scientists cannot make these synthetic forms of the vitamin the only source of vitamin A in the body of young, growing animals. The animals will be stunted and unhealthy. But, just to keep the epithelial cells healthy, **the synthetic forms of vitamin A, called retinoids, are more likely to do the job of preventing cancer, since they can be given in much larger doses than the natural vitamin A.**

Hamsters, for example, cannot take even half as much natural vitamin A as synthetic retinoids without getting sick.

This is the reason the synthetic forms (called retinoic acid) are used in experiments on cancer. Dr. Sporn calls these forms of vitamin A "drugs" and says they should be used just as preventive drugs, to shield us against cancer in those parts of the body where epithelial cells predominate.

Dr. Sporn says, in his conclusion, **"Vitamin A and its synthetic analogs (retinoids) have been successfully used to prevent cancer of the skin, lung, bladder and breast in experimental animals.** This is a pharmacological (drug) approach to prevention of cancer by enhancement of intrinsic epithelial defense mechanism. Synthetic retinoids are definitely superior for this purpose."

This is very cheering news for two reasons. First a spokesman of the National Cancer Institute is talking about *prevention* of cancer rather than cure. And, secondly, he is talking of using a harmless form of a vitamin in order to prevent cancer. This is such a drastic change from the usual NCI pronouncements that we must be greatly cheered by it.

How might such "drugs" as these be used in human beings? Let's say somebody has already developed skin cancer and the cancer has been removed by surgery. It is unlikely that such a cancer would return or that it will provoke other cancers in other parts of the body. But the person who has already developed a cancer on one epithelial tissue—the skin—should be protected from developing a cancer in the bladder, say, or the lungs. So the synthetic forms of vitamin A, the retinoids, could be given to such an individual to give him or her harmless protection against any further cancers in those parts of the body where vitamin A controls cell division—the skin and the linings of all body openings. So the bladder cancer or the lung cancer could be prevented.

We don't know whether the NCI will be able to convince the medical establishment that a vitamin is better medicine than toxic drugs. The retinoids cannot be patented, so nobody can make as much money selling them to doctors as the drug companies make selling drugs that destroy the patient while they destroy the invading cancer. We hope the retinoids are a major step forward to a time when all cancer will be prevented by judicious use of vitamins and excellent diets. We think this is quite possible right now, without any further research.

National Observer, April 16, 1977, commenting on the NCI research, states: "Researchers learned more than 50 years ago that vitamin A (the real one, remember, not the synthetic one) played some role in controlling the growth of epithelial cells—the cells that form the linings of such organs as the lungs, breast, colon, rectum, pancreas, bladder and esophagus—and played some role in the development of epithelial cancers. If the vitamin is missing, normal cell differentiation and maturing doesn't occur."

Science, the publication of the American Association for the Advancement of Science, devoted a page in its December 27, 1974 issue to the unchallengeable fact that **vitamin A prevents cancer, in both laboratory animals and human beings**. A number of papers read at a symposium on the subject in November, 1974 clearly showed that such is the case. No one knows why or how this occurs, since, it seems, biologists have really very little information on just what vitamin A does in the body and how it does it.

But two scientists from the National Cancer Institute in Washington reported at the symposium that when they applied known cancer-causing substances to parts of the breathing apparatus of animals, much more damage was done to those animals which had been deficient in vitamin A.

Two scientists from Massachusetts Institute of Technology reported that when laboratory rats are given cancer-causing substances which exist in certain fungi that grow on food, there were fewer colon cancers among those rats which got plenty of vitamin A.

Another researcher has found, he said, that in animals who are not at all deficient in vitamin A giving more of the vitamin than they are getting will protect them against cancer of the respiratory tract.

A scientist at the Southern Research Institute at Birmingham, Alabama reported at the symposium that when he applied vitamin A to mice prostate glands he could prevent the cancer that would be expected to follow exposure to certain cancer-causing chemicals. And even if he gave the vitamin A *after* he had exposed the glands to the carcinogens, cancers were prevented.

Another scientist at the same institute tested vitamin A in relation to liver and lung cancer. **He found that vitamin A prevented the formation of a cancer-causing substance from a benzene product.** Both liver and lungs of the animals were protected.

A scientist at the Oak Ridge National Laboratory showed that **vitamin A can reduce the incidence of lung cancers produced by still another cancer-causing compound.** A cancer researcher at the Illinois Institute of Technology reported that giving one form of vitamin A to hamsters prevents cancers that would otherwise be caused by another benzene compound.

And even after the cells have been transformed into pre-cancerous cells, administration of vitamin A can reverse the change and prevent the cancers in some cases, according to a Hoffman-LaRoche scientist, who prevented the formation of one kind of cancer in rats which had been exposed to a substance known to cause this kind of cancer. Their cells had already been starting to form cancers when the vitamin was given.

A Swiss scientist reported that he has prevented certain kinds of cancer in both mice and human beings, after they have been exposed to cancer-causing substances. The evidence appears to be quite substantial and authoritative. There seems to be no doubt. And these reports follow many earlier reports along these same lines.

In spite of all this evidence which, one would suppose, any dedicated lover of humanity would want to shout to the high heavens, the *Science* writer says that unfortunately nobody knows just how or why the vitamin works these miracles.

And apparently in the present state of science and research it is quite impossible for any responsible scientist to urge the immediate publication of these facts so that everyone can benefit from them. No, indeed. First, our learned scientists must probe and tinker, must spend many more years and who knows how many millions of dollars designing more and more experiments before anyone will dare to make the simple statement that it might be a good idea to make sure you are getting enough vitamin A!

Indeed, says *Science*, "Although these results are very encouraging, they are also somewhat distressing, for they hold the potential to provoke a new nutritional fad that could far outstrip those associated with vitamin C and E." Unlike C and E, the writer goes on, "vitamin A is highly toxic at doses slightly higher than the minimum daily requirement." Where he got this information is anybody's guess. One can only assume he made it up as most other careless writers have done since the FDA has proclaimed its vendetta against vitamin A.

At the above-named symposium, one speaker, Barbara Underwood of Pennsylvania State University, announced that **as many as 30 per cent of our population have below-average concentrations of vitamin A in their livers, suggesting that we are deficient in vitamin A.** As we have mentioned in this book, other surveys have also indicated low levels of vitamin A in many people.

According to research at the Massachusetts Institute of Technology, **vitamin A may help to prevent lung cancers and other cancers caused by environmental pollutants.** It appears as well that a deficiency in this vitamin may increase the risk of colon cancer. If the epithelial cells do not have enough of this essential vitamin to maintain their health, they are likely to succumb to cancer, according to Dr. Paul M. Newberne.

Dr. Newberne tells us that anyone can achieve a "normal" amount of vitamin A through a balanced diet which includes yellow and dark green vegetables and liver. But Dr.

Newberne apparently doesn't know many people who follow such a diet, for he goes on to say that an estimated one out of every four Americans is deficient in vitamin A, which might, of course, have a great deal to do with the fact that cancer takes more American lives than any disease except heart disease.

There is abundant evidence available, according to the *British Medical Journal*, that **vitamin A deficiency predisposes to cancers of "squamous" epithelial cells**—that is, the flat, thin cells that form the linings of organs. And adequate levels of vitamin A at meals and in supplements protect against such cancers over a lifetime. The natural vitamin A which is stored in the livers of animals protects them against cancer of these cells, even when the animals have not been given much vitamin A, and even when they are exposed to potent cancer-causing chemicals.

In 1975, a researcher showed that there is a relation between lung cancer and low intake of vitamin A which suggested that **smokers might protect themselves against lung cancer by increasing their intake of vitamin A**. The *British Medical Journal* editorial states that these earlier researches may have sparked the National Cancer Institute decision to test retinoids. Says the *BMJ*, "A wealth of experimental evidence suggests that this hope (of preventing cancer) is not as unreasonable as it might appear, and we may therefore await the outcome of the trial with cautious optimism."

Incidentally, *Nutrition Reviews*, September, 1976, reviews the interesting **relationship between vitamin C and vitamin A in regard to good health**, expecially the health of the adrenal glands which help to protect us from stress. Most animals, except human beings, make their own vitamin C in their livers in very large amounts. Researchers have found that animals who are deficient in vitamin A are somehow unable to manufacture enough vitamin C to protect their adrenal glands from exhaustion under stress. By giving these animals vitamin C, scientists could maintain good health.

It seems reasonable to suppose that human beings, unable to make their own vitamin C, also suffer from exhaustion of the adrenal glands when they are not getting enough vitamin A. Could this not be a cause of cancer, since cancer is certainly a form of stress? The adrenals help to protect us from stress. Now if the human being who is not getting enough vitamin A is also not getting enough vitamin C, it seems certain the whole mechanism might break down, doesn't it? Heavy smokers, for example, are chronically short on vitamin C. The vitamin detoxifies the ill effects of the nicotine and is used up in the process. So the heavy smoker who gets almost no vitamin A has two strikes against him or her.

Three Swiss physicians reported on a test of **vitamin A used against leukoplakia and basal cell carcinoma (cancer) of the skin**. Leukoplakia is a pre-cancerous condition of the mouth and throat. The abstract of their article in *Schweizerische Medizinische Wochenschrift*, July 17, 1971, does not indicate how much vitamin A they gave. It was probably quite large doses.

Of the 24 patients studied, "a therapeutic result" was achieved in 11 who had leukoplakia and short-term remissions were observed in two patients with skin cancer. There were no unpleasant side effects, except that several of the patients complained of headaches.

The cancer cells of all patients who were treated showed changes when the vitamin A was given, and the changes depended upon how much of the vitamin was given. We assume this means that when the dosage was decreased, the cells began to look unhealthy again.

Three articles on vitamin A and its effect on various aspects of cancer therapy are of interest. They assume added importance because they appear in the *Journal of the National Cancer Institute*. This is a Washington-based, government-sponsored organization which should, we believe, be dedicated to the prevention of cancer in any conceivable manner. Instead, they deal mostly with research relating to "cures" and laboratory methods. So it is heartening when one finds anything in their journal which seems to be related to prevention of cancer. Certainly anything pertaining to vitamins would be in this area.

In the first article (March, 1972), six scientists described their discovery that **vitamin A deficiency produces the same condition in the respiratory tract of the hamster as a certain cancer-causing chemical produces**. In other words, a diagnostician examining such an animal would not be able to tell whether the condition he found was due to simple lack of vitamin A or to exposure to a cancer-causing compound.

Did you ever read in any magazine of general circulation that vitamin A deficiency may be a forerunner of cancer, at least in those parts of us relating to breathing—throat, trachea, lungs? Yet that is what this bit of research seems to show, wouldn't you say? A condition which looks like cancer and appears to be cancerous when examined in a laboratory can be caused either by a lack of vitamin A or by a chemical known to cause cancer.

One of the scientists working on this research, Dr. Umberto Saffiotti, announced several years ago that **plenty of vitamin A will protect animals (and presumably human beings) from some of the terribly toxic, cancer-producing chemicals in urban air pollution.** Protect them from possible lung cancer, that is.

In the second article, three Texas doctors report on some experimental radiation to control a cancer. They found that, **if they were injecting vitamin A at the same time, they could reduce by 15 to 20 per cent the radiation needed to stop growth of a certain kind of cancer.** Most of the article deals with the methods they used and their thinking in regard to why this protection should take place.

Finally, they say, "If the effectiveness of a radiation dose to a human tumor could be increased by 15 to 20 per cent without influencing damage to normal tissues, the results of clinical radiotherapy would greatly improve." Although the circumstances of the tumor were not the same as they would be in a human case of cancer, the authors say, "the use of vitamin A ... with therapy of various animal tumors and normal tissues seems worthy of further studies."

It certainly seems so. Radiation is, of course, a terribly dangerous procedure. It must be controlled in such a way that only the cancerous cells are irradiated. This must be done without harming healthy cells. If the simple, easy, inexpensive administration of vitamin A beforehand could lessen the danger of this treatment 15 to 20 per cent, what in heaven's name are we waiting for? **Why isn't vitamin A being used in every cancer treatment center in the world where radiation is used?**

Furthermore, the environmental radioactivity of our world is increasing at a rapid rate. As more and more radioactive substances are used, as nuclear power plants spring up all over the world, releasing their toxic by-products into air and water, isn't it possible that vitamin A could help to protect us against the harm we will certainly face eventually from this increasing contamination? And this contamination is not just from the environment. It may come from sources closer to home, such as in some microwave ovens.

The third article is from the November, 1971 issue of the *International Journal of Vitamin and Nutrition Research*. It tells the dismal story of how little prepared are some of the most vulnerable people to meet any situation which requires plenty of vitamin A for protection. Old folks are always at a special disadvantage. Cancer takes a high toll in these age brackets. Cells are worn out. Resistance is low. Nutrition is usually very inadequate. Meals are skimpy and planned with little attention to vitamin needs.

So vitamin A supplements in ample amounts would seem to be essential for their good health. Yet every survey done, especially among older people, shows that many of them are getting less than recommended amounts of vitamin A, in some cases far less.

The *Journal* article reports on studies of the vitamin A content of food in three old age homes. They happen to be in Switzerland, but old age homes are the same the world around, those in our country included. All of the 38 subjects studied were getting less than 85 per cent of the recommended amount of vitamin A which is 5,000 units daily. Four of the people studied were getting less than 1,250 units daily. In only one home did the diet which was served provide enough vitamin A. In the other two it did not. In any case, most of the old folks refused to eat considerable amounts of their meals, so they did not get even the less-than-recommended amounts of vitamin A that were offered to them.

The study included vitamin C as well, and here the deficiency figures are horrifying. All of the subjects were getting less than 75 per cent of the recommended 55 to 60 milligrams of vitamin C. Since then, the recommended daily dietary allowance for vitamin C has been lowered to 45 milligrams. Isn't that hard to believe? At any rate, in one home the average intake of vitamin C reached only 8 milligrams during the entire week. Twelve of these old people ate less than one milligram of vitamin C on certain days, and they refused up to 87 per cent of whatever vitamin C was offered.

Old people suffer from many complaints which are likely to involve nothing more or less than lack of vitamins. They are highly susceptible to infections (lack of vitamin A and vitamin C). They have trouble with eyes and ears, digestive tracts and elimination. Vitamins in ample amounts can help prevent all these. Their bones, joints and muscles ache—a sure symptom of scurvy which is the disease of vitamin C deficiency. And certainly anyone getting as little vitamin C as these folks were getting is on the very edge of scurvy or perhaps has a full-blown case of scurvy which has just not been diagnosed.

And what of the frightful risk of cancer to which these old

people are exposed when they are eating not even a tiny fraction of the amount of vitamin A and C which is recommended for perfectly healthy adults? Old age is stress. The diseases of old age are a form of stress. **Under stress our bodies need more of all vitamins, but especially vitamin A and C.**

Getting back to **radiation**, two startling revelations by the FDA in May, 1976 were accepted apparently without a murmur by the American public, conditioned as it is to stories of dire catastrophes which will be their daily lot from now on. Some false teeth are radioactive, said the FDA, adding that they may recommend to the Nuclear Regulatory Commission that the permitted levels of uranium in dentures should be reduced. Uranium is used to give natural fluorescence and coloring to porcelain teeth in dentures.

At present the official limit of uranium is 500 parts per million which delivers about 1.5 rem of beta radiation per year—the limit for human beings, according to *Chemical and Engineering News*, May 10, 1976. Since dentures actually contain only about half this amount, said FDA, present radiation from dentures does not constitute a hazard to health. But just the same the official limit should probably be lowered.

And the FDA revealed in May, 1976 that an estimated one tenth of all Americans are wearing eye glasses that are radioactive. Once again, said the FDA spokesman, the amount of radioactivity is "low" and "probably not harmful." One out of every two Americans wears prescription lens glasses.

Both the FDA and the Nuclear Regulatory Commission said they have not uncovered a single case of an American who has suffered any health damage as a result of this constant bombardment by radioactive rays from eye glasses.

The Atomic Energy Commission, the previous nuclear regulatory agency, stated some time ago in a study released only recently, "It is not possible to state unequivocally that there is zero risk to the eye. But the limited information available suggests that the risk to the public is very low, if any, at the levels of radiation observed in our measurements."

Just the same, the FDA, ever mindful of public health even at this late date, asked the Optical Manufacturers Association more than two years ago to agree on new standards that would lower the amount of radioactivity in eye glasses to "as low a level as practicable." The Association agreed and issued guidelines to their industry.

Is there anything you can do? It is doubtful that your dentist or optometrist can tell you whether or not your dentures or eye glasses are radioactive, although you can certainly ask. Please do not write to us as we have no way of knowing either. About the only thing that we can suggest is that you maintain a strong nutritional defense against the possibility of getting cancer. That means eating properly and taking your supplements daily. It means taking special care of your teeth, if you still have them, so as to hopefully avoid getting dentures. And it also means keeping your eyes as healthy as possible so that you may not need glasses.

The radioactivity in spectacles was found when the U. S. Army discovered that sniperscopes they were releasing to Army surplus stores were radioactive. Since AEC regulations forbid selling as surplus any radioactive materials, they investigated and found that the radioactivity was coming from traces of thorium and uranium present in zirconium oxides used to give the glass higher resolving powers.

They looked through more stuff being sold as surplus and found lots of radioactive sunglasses. (It is not immediately apparent just how it happens that many pairs of sunglasses stocked by the Army and paid for, of course, out of taxpayers' money, happen to have become "surplus." Aren't soldiers still wearing sunglasses?) Anyway, studying 441 samples of glass used to make eye glasses, the AEC found that 90 of them were emitting more than 20 atomic disintegrations per minute for each gram of glass. Seven of the samples emitted more than 50 disintegrations. Four showed more than 100 disintegrations. One sample was emitting 359 disintegrations per minute.

The AEC describes as "contaminated" anything above 20 disintegrations per minute. According to the *Washington Post* for May 18, 1976, "most of the radiation discharged by the contaminants was found to be alpha radiation which never penetrates the eye below the cornea. None the less, the AEC said a person wearing contaminated eye glasses 16 hours a day would receive an annual dose of radiation eight times that permitted by law."

The harm done by radiation is cumulative. That is, the more radiation you receive during a lifetime the greater the danger of cancer, of susceptibility to many other degenerative diseases, or of genetic damage to offspring. You already receive radiation from cosmic rays and other radioactive elements called "background radiation." Many experts believe that most genetically-caused defects down through the ages were the result of this background radiation *alone.*

Now, because of human tinkering with radioactive substances, you are being bombarded with far more radioactivity than that. And it comes from many sources, including the remnants of radioactive fallout from bombs, as we know. X-rays contribute immense doses of radiation. Yet they are used almost as casually as tongue depressors in some medical clinics. Experts who estimate the "permissible doses" for a lifetime deal only in one item or another—never the sum total of all the radiation you receive during a lifetime.

When the Chinese set off a nuclear bomb in 1977, the radioactive fallout eventually reached a wide strip of area along the Eastern United States. At least one researcher blamed the fallout for the deaths of a number of infants, although this has been disputed.

At any rate, the annual dose of radiation from eye glasses which is eight times that permitted by law does not take into account all the other sources of radiation to which you are exposed. If you have had long series of X-rays, you have undoubtedly had far more than the "permissible dose" just from that source alone. But the total damage done is the cumulative amount of radiation you receive over a lifetime. And there is no way to determine whether a cancer is caused by radiation or by some other harmful element in our environment. So we will never know how many cancers may finally result from the uranium in eye glasses and dentures.

Apparently there is no reason except carelessness why either of these should contain radioactive substances. In the case of dentures the reason for using the uranium is cosmetic only—so the teeth will look like real teeth! And for this you have been exposed to atomic radiation every moment that these dentures or other dental fixtures are in your mouth. No one told you. You were simply forced to assume this risk whether you wanted to or not.

Most wearers of dentures and eye glasses are older folks— the very people who have already accumulated perhaps far more than the "permissible" limits of radiation throughout their lifetime, the very people who are least able to bear the burden of still further radiation.

Patients with cancer should be given vitamin supplements, says *Medical World News* soberly, reporting on observations of two Scots physicians who studied the vitamin C status of 50 cancer patients. They found that almost all had vitamin C levels that were low and 30 of them had "very low" levels. Most of them were just not getting "enough" vitamin C in their diets to prevent scurvy, said the two physicians. So, to prevent scurvy, they went on, these folks should be given vitamin C supplements.

While on the subject of vitamin C, two articles co-authored by Dr. Linus Pauling question whether vitamin C may not be a very helpful therapy for cancer victims. An article in *Chemical and Biological Interactions*, 9 (4), 273-283, 1974, states that resistance to cancer may be enhanced by vitamin C. The two authors, Dr. Pauling and Dr. Ewan Cameron, state also that the potential value of vitamin C in the supportive therapy of cancer is a matter for urgent study. The vitamin offers a promise of general improvement in the results of cancer treatment when standard methods of treatment are being used.

A recent study showed that people who work in beauty parlors have a 10 times greater chance of dying from lung cancer than people in other occupations. Three Berkeley, California physicians made this announcement in July, 1975. The study covered only one county in California including 3,000 beauticians. But the scientists said they believed it to be a representative figure for the entire country. Others pointed out that the lung cancer figures may simply mean that beauticians smoke more than other people or that they are exposed to more environmental poisons of other kinds than other people.

If, indeed, this study ties in with other laboratory studies **incriminating hair dyes as cancer-causing chemicals,** one might ask why hair dyes should cause lung cancer rather than scalp cancer or skin cancer. No one knows the answer to this one. But it seems apparent that employees of beauty parlors are exposed all day to cigarette smoke in a small, badly ventilated area in which they are also in close, daily contact with countless other cosmetic preparations, any one of which may be the offending agent. Or, what is more likely, perhaps it is the sum total of all these environmental chemicals which dooms the beautician to cancer at much higher rate of incidence. Hair sprays are sprayed from aerosol cans. The beautician's hands are almost eternally deep in some kind of dye or other cosmetic preparations. Surely the assault of all these toxins over a lifetime must have a deleterious effect. It seems to us that someone should make a definitive and meaningful study soon. Meanwhile, we recommend no hair dyes at all and only those cosmetics for both hair and skin which are available at your health food store.

Still another experiment has been reported demonstrating **the power of vitamin A to prevent cancer.** As reported in *Science*, three scientists at the National Cancer Institute in

Bethesda, Maryland tell us that it has been known for a long time that certain kinds of cancers are prevented when enough vitamin A is given. Vitamin A has been found to be powerful against cancers caused by certain viruses and against cancers caused by chemicals known to cause cancer, as we have noted.

In the most dramatic of such experiments, mice were protected from air pollutants when they were given vitamin A. These are the same air pollutants to which all of us are exposed when we go into or live in a city or anywhere near traffic lanes or industries where air pollution is a problem. Animals not getting vitamin A develop cancer routinely. Those which are given vitamin A do not.

But laboratory scientists have ways of giving cancer to animals aside from exposing them to cancer-causing substances. They transplant or graft the cancers on to the animal. In this case they used laboratory mice in which they transplanted a certain kind of tumor—a murine melanoma. Before transplanting the tumors, they had given quite large doses of vitamin A to half the mice. It was given in their drinking water. The other half of the mice got plain drinking water.

After two weeks of giving the vitamin, the cancerous cells were injected in varying numbers. In one experiment, 17 per cent of the vitamin A-treated animals injected with cancer cells developed cancers, compared with 100 per cent of the untreated animals. At another dosage, 83 per cent of the untreated animals got cancer while only 58 per cent of those which got vitamin A developed tumors.

In other tests, the scientists injected the vitamin A rather than giving it by mouth. Five per cent of the injected animals got cancer, while 76 per cent of those unprotected by vitamin A got cancer. In addition, the tumors of the vitamin A-treated group were much smaller than those of the animals which got no vitamin. In one of the tests where a large amount of a particularly virulent cancer was transplanted, it took 15,000 units of vitamin A over a short period of time to protect the

84

animals against the cancers which developed, as expected, in the group not getting vitamin A. This is an extremely large amount of vitamin A for an animal the size of a mouse.

They do not know, say these scientists, why or how vitamin A protects against this kind of tumor when it is transplanted or injected. They think it has something to do with immunity systems—that is, the vitamin A helps the body to develop immunity against the tumor.

The New York Times for March 28, 1975 published **a list of chemicals which have been authoritatively linked to cancer in human beings.** The list included aflatoxin which may cause liver cancer; 4-Aminobiphenyl which may cause bladder cancer; arsenic compounds which may cause skin and lung cancer; asbestos which may cause lung and digestive cancer; auramine which may cause bladder cancer; benzene which may cause bone marrow cancer; benzidine which may cause bladder cancer; Bis (chloromethyl ether) which may cause lung cancer; cadmium which may cause prostate cancer; chromium in chromate-producing industries which may produce lung cancer; hematite which may cause lung cancer; naphthylamine which may cause bladder cancer; nickel in nickel-refining which may cause nasal or lung cancer; soot and tars which may cause bladder cancer; stilbestrol which may cause vaginal and uterine cancer and vinyl chloride which may cause liver, brain or lung cancer.

The New York Academy of Sciences has decided to translate into layman's language a four-day symposium on occupational cancer. Dr. Sidney Wolfe of the Health Research Group (affiliated with Ralph Nader) has offered to do the "translation" into words and ideas the non-scientists can understand. It seems that workers, their unions and health organizations do not take action sooner on cancer-causing chemicals because they just do not have enough information about the hazards involved.

But, of course, in the case of many of the above chemicals, all of us are exposed almost continually in our daily lives: to asbestos, for instance, and arsenic in pesticides, soots and tars from charred meats and coal tar food additives, stilbestrol in the DES which farmers use in meat and which doctors give as "morning-after" birth control pills. To say nothing of polyvinyl chloride which is, of course, the plastic wrap which wraps everything you buy at a supermarket. Apparently no one has ever done any research to see how much of it migrates into the food.

On April 18, 1975 the Environmental Protection Agency announced that they had found **potential cancer-causing agents in the drinking water of all of the 79 cities in the country which they had tested.** No one knows how much water one must drink in order to fall prey to cancer caused by the small amounts of such chemicals in the water supply. Chlorine, used to kill water-borne bacteria, seems to be the chief villain. The public has been told for many years that this water purifying agent is perfectly harmless, even though no one ever did any tests to prove that it is. Our waterworks people just went right on using it and assuring us that it was safe.

Now experts have discovered that **chlorine in the water combines with other chemicals to form carcinogens.** These other chemicals may come from sewage discharges, from water treatment processes, from industrial discharges and from runoff from urban areas and farms.

Says the *Washington Post*, "In addition to the 79 water systems checked only for these six compounds, the EPA released reports of extensive testing it has done in five cities. The results in those areas—Philadelphia, Miami, Cincinnati, Seattle and Ottumwa—are similar to those found in New Orleans. Both Cincinnati and Philadelphia had 36 substances in their water. Miami had 35." Both these two cities also had dieldrin in their water—a pesticide known to cause cancer, and vinyl chloride, the chemical from which plastic is made.

The *Washington Post* asked Dr. Umberto Saffiotti of the National Cancer Institute for his opinion of the hazards faced by people who drink this water. He said, "Our present position is that we have no methodology we can rely on to determine safe levels of carcinogens." Age and susceptibility, the air we breathe, the food we eat—all these are variables. "We suspect that any small insults will add up with others to make the level in another. All we can say is that less exposure is better than more exposure," he added.

On April 27, 1975 the National Cancer Institute announced that a nationwide survey provided information that seems to show that **some kinds of cancer predominate in areas of the country where certain industries are congregated.** Higher than normal death rates from bladder cancer were found in New Jersey, in urban areas around the Great Lakes and in rural New York and New England. Industries located there include chemical plants and industries involved with wood products, stone, clay and glass. High rates of lung cancer were found along the Gulf Coast and the Southeast Atlantic coast. Kidney cancers were found most prevalent in rural Wisconsin, Minnesota and the Dakotas.

A study done by the Labor Department concluded that **one out of every four workers in industry has a disease related to his occupation.** And 89 per cent of these are not reported, as required, to the Labor Department. Some of the diseases are: chronic respiratory disease, loss of hearing due to noise, cataracts from infra-red radiation and lead in the blood. Workers were not closely studied, with thorough physical examinations. If such investigations had been done it is believed that even more illness would have come to light. Said a spokesman, "Yet despite the limited nature of the investigation, the high incidence of disease is appalling." On a national scale the incidence of work-related disease is probably about 21 million workers. Many more office workers are exposed to potential carcinogens every day in the multitude of chemicals that are used on office machines, typewriter ribbons, type-cleaning fluids, typing eraser devices, copy machine chemicals, etc.

On April 26, 1975 a National Cancer Institute study revealed that a chemical used in metal industries has been found to cause cancer in the livers and other organs of laboratory animals. This is trichloroethylene, closely related to polyvinyl chloride. More than 600 million pounds of this new chemical are produced every year for use in industry. It is a degreasing agent in the metal industry and solvent and dry cleaning agent in the clothing industry. It is also used in food processing—formerly used to remove caffeine from coffee and to isolate spice resins.

Dr. Umberto Saffiotti made the announcement because, he said, it may help people to protect themselves from a cancer hazard. Many workers who are occupationally exposed to this chemical are also exposed to many other potentially dangerous chemicals which may, of course, greatly increase the risk. The Food and Drug Administration allows up to 10 parts per million of this solvent in instant decaffeinated coffee and up to 25 parts per million in ground decaf. Since this announcement was made, it is believed that the coffee industry has switched to another chemical to remove caffeine from coffee.

Metal workers and garage attendants get wider exposure than any of the rest of us, when they hover over large vats of the degreasing solvent to dip pieces of greasy metal into it.

The Cancer Institute tested on animals amounts of this chemical that were not inappropriate in comparison to human exposure. Said Dr. Saffiotti, "The preliminary results of these tests indicate that it is highly likely that this chemical is carcinogenic."

On March 29, 1975, *The National Observer* printed the story of a student wearing a watch with a luminous dial. Suspicious of a shadow on the dial, he had it tested for **radioactivity** and found that it emitted radiation equal to 100 times that of a typical chest X-ray. Little more than four hours of direct body contact with the crystal could give the wearer as much radiation as scientists consider permissible for an entire year! The same man had used a similar pocket watch for six months. Both watches were bought from an army surplus store in West Germany. The army refuses to believe that the watches can be hazardous, although they have withdrawn them from sale. *The Observer* article tells us that there is no federal regulation of substances that are "naturally" radioactive like radium. Laws to regulate the availability of such materials are left to the states.

"With the exception of a New York City ordinance against making radium watches, there apparently are no laws against the import or manufacture of radium-painted consumer products," says the newspaper. At least 600,000 radium-dial clocks were sold throughout the United States during a three-year period ending in January, 1974, and an untold number of old clocks and watches and other articles remain in use.

The professor who measured the amount of radiation from the original wristwatch told his student that, "If the watch is worn for any length of time, cancer of the colon and stomach will probably result. **Genetic damage is also a real threat since most of the men who purchased these watches are young and not through procreating.**"

Dr. Saffiotti, who made the ominous announcements about the cancer-causing solvent and the hazards of drinking water, is the same National Cancer Institute scientist who, over 10 years ago, told the public on the front page of *The New York Times* about Institute tests which had shown that vitamin A gives complete protection to animals exposed to certain cancer-causing substances. None of the animals in the test was deficient in vitamin A. None of them was given too much of it. But those animals which were given sizable supplements of vitamin A did not get cancer from the carcinogens to which they were exposed, while other animals which did not get the supplements all got cancer.

At the time Dr. Saffiotti warned that private citizens should not begin to take vitamin A or eat a lot of carrots (which contain it) because that might be harmful! True, it didn't harm the animals. Instead it protected them from harm. But human beings? It's apparently not the job of the National Cancer Institute to do much research on ways of preventing cancer and, if a few such experiments slip through, we are immediately warned not to apply them to ourselves. Vitamins are deadly substances is the impression we are carefully given.

At the Ninth International Cancer Congress in 1941, a British scientist, Sir Alexander Haddow, announced that **as many as 80 per cent of all human cancers may be due to environmental causes**. If this is true, he said, "The implications for prevention are immense and exciting." He believes that scientists will be able to eliminate most cancers, even if they never find out what causes cancer. We're sorry that we cannot agree with Haddow.

What he is saying, in essence, is that as soon as we have final irrevocable proof that air pollution, water pollution, chemicals in food, pesticides, drugs, cigarette smoke, radiation and all the other pollutants of our industrial society cause cancer, then all we have to do is to eliminate these hazards and we won't have any more cancer. But what an impossible premise!

Men of good will admit today that these environmental hazards pose serious threats to health. But the job of eliminating them from the world we live in is impossibly immense. No government has made even a token start on such a job. Nor is there any assurance that, with the best will in the world, any government will ever succeed in protecting us from all the hazards to which our present technological society exposes us.

And when a leading scientist finds that we can lessen the threat of cancer in at least some people by taking a bit more of a perfectly wholesome vitamin, the same scientist feels he must warn us most vehemently against this, because he once heard that a few babies given incredibly large doses suffered some transient unpleasant symptoms. We are speaking again about Dr. Saffiotti who first made headlines with the news that vitamin A could be useful in treating some cancers. Then he cautioned against taking too much of the vitamin.

Let's not go over the statistics on air pollution. Everyone knows that the situation is scandalous and is getting steadily worse rather than better. Let's talk about cigarettes instead. All scientists know perfectly well that cigarette smoke causes cancer. Yet Americans of all ages are buying and smoking cigarettes in greater numbers than before. More and more women are smoking, which means that more of them will be succumbing to cancer, emphysema, etc.

At the same time, every survey shows our teenagers, especially teenage girls, eat worse diets than anyone else in the country. Any teenage girl, determined to keep her figure, has probably eliminated from her diet in a mistaken idea of "reducing" most of the foods that might supply her with enough vitamin A—liver, eggs and butter, chiefly. Her liking for carrots and leafy green vegetables is probably minimal. (Who wants to eat rabbit food, and besides they don't serve it at the teenage hangout). Where is the vitamin A in her diet that may help to protect this young woman from cancer?

Meanwhile, the American Cancer Society duly presents its yearly figures: **One American in every four will eventually have cancer.** But, we are told, don't take any vitamin A to possibly prevent cancer, because a few people have taken too much. Wouldn't it seem more altruistic as well as more practical for both the American Cancer Society and Dr. Saffiotti to recommend passing a law to make it mandatory for every smoker and everyone who is exposed to cigarette smoke at work or at home to take a vitamin A supplement every day of his life? What should be meant by "preventive medicine," if not something like this?

Meanwhile, *Medical World News* for September 6, 1976 reported that a drug company scientist in Switzerland obtained **excellent results using several "cousins" of vitamin A on skin conditions that defied all other kinds of treatment.** They involved precancerous and cancerous skin conditions.

Dr. H. Mayer used retinoic acid (the vitamin A cousin) on 60 patients with actinic keratosis (a pre-cancerous condition) and on 16 others with basal cell carcinoma. In the first group, 40 per cent had complete regression and 45 per cent partial regression. In the second group, 31 per cent had complete regression and 63 per cent had partial regression.

He also treated 33 patients with bladder cancers. A one per cent solution of the same substance instilled directly into the patient's bladder every day for 20 days produced complete or partial regression for 22 patients. The researchers working with these "drugs", as they call them, emphasize that much more work must be done but the vitamin A "cousins offer some promise", according to a spokesman of the National Cancer Institute.

We do not tell you horror stories about cancer to frighten you into withdrawing from society and going to live on an isolated island. We believe—and we have presented much scientific evidence to confirm our belief—that you can protect yourself from cancer by: 1) Avoiding all exposure to carcinogens that you can possibly avoid. This means checking carefully on occupational hazards. Work through your union or public health officials to eliminate such hazards. 2) Don't buy foods or household equipment of any kind which is even suspected of being harmful. Buy only fresh, unprocessed foods and rely mostly on staples at your health food store where every effort is made to keep every item free from contaminants. 3) Don't use suspect cosmetics like hair dyes and conditioners. Don't use pesticides or herbicides. Avoid as much as possible office chemicals that might be carcinogenic. Get as little exposure as possible to known air pollutants like car and bus exhaust and incinerator smoke. 4) Use the best possible diet and diet supplements as weapons against cancer and every other degenerative disease. 5) Don't smoke. Avoid if possible all public places where a lot of smokers congregate. Work for more no-smoking areas in your office and city.

If you are exposed to any chemicals or pollutants that are known to cause cancer, you need more vitamin A than someone not so exposed. Also increase your vitamin C intake. This means that city dwellers automatically need more vitamin A, generally speaking, than country dwellers, for they must continually breathe the polluted city air. Of course, we have indicated in this chapter that some rural areas are heavily polluted by industries. If you smoke, your needs for vitamin A are probably much much greater than those of the non-smoker. If you live in a house or work in an office or factory where others smoke, you need more vitamin A than someone not so exposed. The vitamin A, as we have learned, is stored in the liver and is called on by your body to aid in the process of keeping healthy cells developing in lungs, bronchial tubes, throat and mouth.

CHAPTER 7

Vitamin A Protects Against Infections

ALTHOUGH VITAMIN A was discovered 60 odd years ago and its chemical nature has been known over 40 years, there are signs it may have valuable properties not suspected until now, according to *Medical World News* for December 14, 1973. This is not news to any health seeker, for we have been using this vitamin for many years as a shield against many different disorders, including infections.

But now a physician-researcher has tested vitamin A to see if it actually does protect against infections. And he found that it does!

Dr. Benjamin E. Cohen of Massachusetts General Hospital reported on his experiment at a meeting of the American Society of Plastic and Reconstructive Surgeons. Presumably these surgeons would be interested in such information since, in many kinds of surgery, the "immune response" is involved. This is the ability of the body to protect itself against invaders of any kind—bacteria, or foreign proteins.

Dr. Cohen found that **vitamin A strongly stimulated his laboratory animals' "immune response"**—that is, it gave them far more capability to withstand diseases.

The drug cortisone is known to block this immune response. This is one reason why people taking cortisone and related drugs are likely to be much more susceptible to infections than the rest of us. So Dr. Cohen gave cortisone to his laboratory mice along with vitamin A. **He found that the vitamin almost completely prevented the action of the cortisone, thereby protecting the body from infection.**

Then he inoculated germs into the animals to which he had previously given injections of 3,000 units of vitamin A— an immense amount of this vitamin for a creature as small as a mouse. He then injected the mice with a gram-negative bacterium, or a fungus or a gram-positive bacterium. He had another group of "control" animals which got no vitamin A.

In the group of mice infected with gram-negative bacteria the control animals suffered massive invasion of the germs and died of the infection within 24 hours. The mice treated with vitamin A developed severe infection for the first three hours, but by the fifth hour "no more organisms could be cultured from their blood." While the mice which had received no vitamin A were dying, the mice treated with vitamin A were found to have blood "still virtually sterile" so far as the injected germs were concerned.

In the case of the other kind of bacteria and the fungus, **the vitamin A treatment greatly prolonged the animals' survival time,** although they did die eventually from the disease, as the untreated mice did.

Dr. Cohen suggested that **vitamin A should be given to patients who are being treated with cortisone and related drugs,** for it will apparently greatly help to protect them from infections. Other researchers have used vitamin A, he says, to reduce the incidence of digestive tract stress in patients suffering from severe trauma, burns or the aftermath of surgery. Dr. Cohen thinks the vitamin should be used to protect burned patients from infection.

He also thinks, he says, that "**vitamin A could play a significant part in cancer therapy** if further studies of its use with BCG support preliminary findings with mice" given a certain kind of cancer (BCG is a vaccine). "In our first couple of experiments we looked at the effects of vitamin A with BCG, compared with BCG alone, on susceptibility to tumor inoculum," said Dr. Cohen. "We found that animals receiving both vitamin A and BCG had a lower incidence of tumors than those getting BCG alone."

One important role of vitamin A is, as scientists know, to protect the integrity of the linings of things in the body—the lining of the digestive tract, the lungs, the eliminative tract, the eyes, ears, nose, throat, the reproductive tract and so on. There have been other research projects showing that it can also protect against cancer, as we see in another chapter in this book.

CHAPTER 8

Dr. Fred Klenner
Speaks Out
on Vitamin A

DURING THE HEIGHT of the controversy, in which the Food and Drug Administration attempted to restrict to 10,000 International Units the amount of vitamin A which can be sold in one tablet or capsule, Dr. Linus Pauling, the two-time Nobel Prize winner discussed the foolishness of such a regulation.

In *Medical Tribune*, Dr. Fred Klenner of Reidsville, North Carolina, paid tribute to Dr. Pauling's ideas, as follows:

"The challenge of Dr. Linus Pauling of the proposed limitations on the non-prescription sale of not only vitamin A but also of all vitamins should be applauded by all physicians. These proposed 'safety' regulations by the Food and Drug Administration would indeed limit the freedom of the people since each individual has the inalienable right to make his own decision regarding his own person.

"As Dr. Pauling stated, **there is very little chance of damage to humans from ingesting vitamin A.** I have one patient with ichthyosis (a skin disease) who has taken 200,000 units of vitamin A daily for over 10 years just to keep his skin within normal texture limits. No toxicity. I have taken from 75,000 units of vitamin A up to 150,000 units daily for the past 25 years. No toxicity.

"I recommend to my patients who drive to take at least 50,000 units of vitamin A daily to improve their night vision. Many traffic deaths could be averted by taking not only vitamin A but also vitamin B1 (200 milligrams) and vitamin C (2,000 milligrams) every hundred miles of driving.

"I suggest that Dr. Charles Edwards (then FDA Commissioner) use the office of the Food and Drug Administration to remove the many known carcinogenic agents (cancer-causing chemicals) from the food they allow us to eat."

Dr. Klenner's reference to his patient with the scaly skin condition, ichthyosis, demonstrates that individual requirements for vitamins may vary many fold. This man obviously must have that much vitamin A just to keep his skin in the same comfortable, reasonably healthy condition the rest of us find normal. Undoubtedly there are many other health conditions in which just the addition of ample amounts of one vitamin or another may mean the difference between good health and lifelong misery.

As we learn in another chapter, night blindness is rather common. As we depend more and more on artificial light to lengthen our days, the effect of that light is to deplete the eyes of the substance—visual purple—which must be there for good vision at night. Vitamin A must be present in ample amounts for this substance to be replenished. Is it any wonder that so many of us see poorly at night, any wonder that so many fatal auto accidents take place at night and at dusk when seeing is difficult?

CHAPTER 9

More News About
Vitamin A

AN INTERESTING COMPLICATION of vitamin A and alcohol was brought out in *Science* for December 6, 1974. It seems that vitamin A is essential for the human male to manufacture sperm. And a certain enzyme is required for converting the vitamin A into a usable form. Alcohol (as in booze) stops the process whereby vitamin A is changed into a usable form to create sperm. So, say the authors, who are from the University of Pittsburgh, it is possible that this vitamin A complication is the reason that some alcoholics are sterile.

Two dramatic developments in regard to vitamin A have been reported from widely separated sources. The National Institutes of Health in Washington, D. C. announced that **vitamin A, applied directly to open sores, rapidly heals them, in patients who are taking cortisone or similar drugs**. These might be patients suffering from rheumatic fever, arthritis, gout or other inflammatory diseases. The drug prevents inflammation, thus easing pain and making things much pleasanter for the victim, although leaving the disease just where it was before drug treatment began.

Following injury, however, inflammation is needed to

trigger the body's natural healing process. This means that open wounds, in people taking cortisone, tend to heal poorly, the risk of infection is much greater and recovery after surgery can be quite lengthy.

So physicians at the University of California Medical Center used vitamin A, applying it directly to the open wounds. Result? Rapid and highly successful healing. Wounds ranged from large non-healing ulcers of the leg to severe infectious wounds on the chest. In several cases, we are told, wounds that had stubbornly resisted healing for weeks healed in a matter of days. **All wounds healed within three weeks.**

The physicians also gave the vitamin orally with some success, but not as great as when it was applied to the wound itself. Then they tried the vitamin on wounds of people not taking cortisone and found that it had no effect. They believe, they say, that the healing effect comes from some unique interaction between the drug with vitamin A, and they think that their discovery may lead to better understanding of the healing process generally.

From *Medical World News* for May 16, 1969 comes word that **vitamin A in ample amounts may prevent stomach cancer** in people who are continuously exposed to cancer-causing substances. American physicians in Korea said that a food which is very popular among Koreans contains a certain fungus, *Aspergillus flavus*, which is known to cause cancer.

Dr. David J. Seel and his associates took detailed diet histories of 70 Koreans suffering from stomach cancer and 70 healthy Koreans. They found that the healthy ones were getting as much as 3,300 units of vitamin A in their daily diets, whereas the cancer victims were getting only an average of 2,853 units. This seems to be quite a small difference, yet the researchers believe it may spell health for one group and tragic illness for the other.

It would seem that the best procedure would be not only to give ample amounts of vitamin A to all Koreans who eat this food item, but also to discourage its use. But it seems to be a traditional staple dish which forms the basis of diet for many extremely poor farmers.

From a hospital in Israel comes word of experiments in which **vitamin A was used to retard the growth and inhibit the induction of benign and malignant tumors in laboratory animals**. This means that applying the vitamin to the skin of the animal prevented cancer from forming when chemicals known to cause cancer were applied. In animals which were already suffering from cancer, growth of the tumor was slowed.

This protective action took place only in the cervix and vagina of the female animals, not on other parts of the body. The experiments were described in *Cancer* magazine.

Injections of vitamin A have consistently improved fertility of cows and weight gain of calves, according to a professor of nutrition at Purdue University. He said that, although the cow's liver is an efficient storehouse of vitamin A, even cows fed on lush grass (rich in vitamin A) during the summer tend to use up these vitamin stores during the winter. Pregnant beef cows are likely to be deficient in vitamin A when they are fed the usual rations.

Note that these are not sick animals, nor animals which are being deliberately made deficient for some experiment. They are the normal, average kind of animal, just as you and I are the average kind of people: Yet when they are being supposedly well-fed (and cows are usually much better fed than most human beings) additional vitamin A can improve their health.

According to a British scientist, vitamins A and E are bound up together in their chemical actions. Says the researcher, writing in *Experimental Eye Research*, "The presence of vitamin E in the diet is of major importance in protecting small quantities of vitamin A from oxidation (that is, destruction by oxygen)."

Vitamin E has a sparing effect on vitamin A and the carotenes. In other words, if you are getting plenty of vitamin E, you can get along with less of the foods rich in vitamin A. This is especially important to keep in mind these days, when most of the vitamin E is removed from our food by refining and processing our cereal grains—the richest source of vitamin E.

A report from an International Conference on Gerontology (the study of old age) on a study done in Budapest, Hungary showed that older people, inactive or bedfast, had low calcium levels in their blood. Giving vitamin preparations containing vitamin A and vitamin D, or vitamin D alone, brought these levels up to normal, although, apparently, no more calcium was given in their diets. Vitamin D is involved in how the body absorbs calcium.

Since we get most of our vitamin D from sunlight, it is reasonable to suppose that people who are bedridden would lack this vitamin. But the doctors found that they could normalize the blood levels of calcium in these older people by giving just vitamin A alone, without the addition of vitamin D, as it comes in fish liver oil. But it was necessary to give three times the amount of vitamin A which is considered to be essential for healthy adults.

"A recent study done at the University of Minnesota in cooperation with USDA's Consumer and Food Economic Research Division, revealed that **although most American children are fairly well fed, their diets may be low in two vitamins important to good health—A and C,**" reported *Food and Home Notes*, the U. S. Department of Agriculture bulletin for August 30, 1967.

"The study showed that children's vitamin A intake was related to their feeling toward dark green and yellow vegetables which are high in vitamin A and the mother's opinion about the importance of serving foods rich in the vitamin. In some cases the mother did not serve them often enough to provide vitamins needed.

"Where the mother had some knowledge of nutrition, and the father had a higher than average income and educational level," the publication goes on, "the families were likely to have a satisfactory intake of vitamin C rich foods. Where the mother had little knowledge of nutrition or the father had a low income, the intake of vitamin C was usually below recommended levels.

"Vitamin A and C are important to health and are problem vitamins all through life since adults seem to follow food patterns established in childhood. Good eating habits are important to good nutrition. . . . "

"Our tests show the startling fact that 70 per cent of our patients are borderline or definitely short on vitamin A," reports Harold F. Hawkins, D.D.S., former Associate Professor of Bacteriology and Preventive Dentistry, College of Dentistry, University of Southern California, in *Applied Nutrition*, a book published by the International College of Applied Nutrition, La Habra, California.

"We have overlooked the fact that this vitamin is not very stable, especially as to heat. A high percentage of vitamin A is injured or destroyed in the pasteurization of milk and butter. Cooking eggs, carrots, spinach and all high sources of this essential factor is detrimental. The prevalence of night blindness and the common cold gives convincing evidence of this deficiency.

Dr. Hawkins goes on to say that it is possible to consume a generous intake of this vitamin and still have low body levels. "We must not forget that vitamin A is a fat soluble vitamin and requires normal fat assimilation. Any impairment in liver function conspires to defeat the body's ability to secure an adequate intake," he added.

CHAPTER 10

It's Not All
That Easy to Get
Enough Vitamin A

THE MURMURS OF alarm which began several years ago over disclosures of widespread vitamin A deficiency are rising to a roar of concern as more and more surveys turn up evidence of shortages in this essential and extremely important vitamin.

At the Western Hemisphere Nutrition Congress, which we discussed earlier in this book, scientists were told by Dr. T. Keith Murray, chief of the Nutrition Research Division of Canada's Food and Drug Directorate, that low intakes of the vitamin and even low blood levels of vitamin A have been found with no physical symptoms apparent. But in one study of children there were significant correlations between low vitamin A status and the incidence of skin and upper respiratory infections and several other symptoms.

"Who knows," asked Dr. Murray, "in a child with blood level deficiencies, how far he is from a frankly deficient state in which symptoms become apparent? Can we not, at the very least, assume that his intake is barely meeting his requirement? If such symptoms are in store for even some of children with low serum levels of vitamin A, we must be concerned."

Then he summarized recent surveys which showed, he said, that **a significant percentage of most age groups in all of North America lack appreciable reserves of vitamin A, and 20 to 30 per cent fail to consume the recommended daily allowance.** Although most North American adults have adequate blood levels of vitamin A, a considerable number of children fall below the acceptable level, with adverse health effects in some of them.

Calling vitamin A deficiency "the subject uppermost in the minds of most delegates to the Congress," *Family Health* for November, 1971 relates once again the alarming statistics showing "the same distressing conclusion: many North Americans are suffering from serious vitamin A deficiencies."

An article in the February, 1973 issue of *Ladies Home Journal* discussed the diets of three First Ladies—Mrs. Richard Nixon, Mrs. Lyndon Johnson and Mrs. Jacqueline Kennedy Onassis. We analyzed their diets in relation to the recommended daily dietary allowances and found that all three of the women were often short on essential nutrients. In the case of vitamin A, only Mrs. Johnson was getting the recommended amount each day. She apparently loves deep green and yellow vegetables, and so her vitamin A intake was 12,450 units—over twice the 5,000 units recommended each day. Mrs. Onassis got only 2,235 units of vitamin A from her diet; Mrs. Nixon even less—1,350 units.

In 1968, the United States Department of Agriculture released the results of an extensive survey conducted by their nutrition experts showing that only about half the families in our country have diets that qualify as "good," let alone excellent. **Vitamin A was one of the nutrients most often found lacking in diets.**

In 1969, the U. S. Public Health Service announced results of a survey of 12,000 individuals conducted by PHS nutritionists whose expertise lies in this field. **They** discovered that 13 per cent of everyone examined [...] less than acceptable levels of vitamin A in their blood.

"I eat carrots every week," you may say, "so I couldn't possibly be short on vitamin A, for everybody knows that carrots are the best source."

It would depend on how many carrots you ate and how well your body is able to convert the carotene from the carrots into vitamin A. It seems likely that you would not be getting sufficient vitamin A, since you are supposed to ingest from 4,000 to 5,000 units daily.

How can you tell if you are short on one or more vitamins? It isn't easy. A quick summary of an article that appeared in the May, 1974 issue of *Geriatrics* seems to be the best answer to this question. The article, by Samuel Dreizen, DDS, M.D., of the University of Texas, deals with older people, but what he says is just as likely to be true of younger folks, if they have been eating unwisely for most of their lives.

Dr. Dreizen points out that the final stages of malnutrition occur only when we have abused our bodies for a considerable time, since we have many compensating mechanisms which help protect us. It is only after all these have been exhausted that the telltale symptoms appear.

"The earliest evidence of malnutrition in the elderly," says Dr. Dreizen, "is a conglomerate of nonspecific complaints that coincide in time with the subclinical phase of nutritive failure." They include such things as: lack of appetite, abdominal discomfort, anxiety, backache, confusion, decreased work output, depression, indigestion, fatigue, headache, insomnia, irritability, lassitude, muscle pain, muscle weakness, nervousness, palpitations (fluttering or noticeable throbbing of the heart), "pins and needles" in arms and legs, lack of ability to concentrate. These symptoms differ from person to person and we must not make the mistake of thinking that all fatigue or all headaches and so on are due to vitamin deficiency.

Of course, vitamin A is only a part of the scheme of things discussed by Dr. Dreizen. **We must have all of the**

Foods High in
Vitamin A

*(The daily recommended minimum
for adults is 5,000 units)*

Food	Units of Vitamin A
Carrots, raw, 1/2 cup	11,000
Sweet potatoes, 1	7,700
Beet greens, 1/2 cup	6,700
Chard, 1/2 cup	8,720
Chicory, 1/2 cup	10,000
Dandelion greens, 1/2 cup	15,170
Endive, 10 stalks	3,000
Kale, cooked, 1/2 cup	8,300
Spinach, cooked, 1/2 cup	11,780
Turnip greens, cooked, 1/2 cup	10,600
Pumpkin, cooked, 1/2 cup	3,400
Cantaloupe, 1/2 small	3,420
Apricots, 6 halves	2,790
Apricots, dry, 8 halves	3,700
Peaches, fresh, 1 large	880
Prunes, dry, 12	1,890
Tomato Juice, 4 oz.	1,050
Liver, beef, fried, 1 serving	53,500
Liver, chicken	32,200
Liverwurst, 1/4 pound	5,750
Eggs, 2	1,140

essential vitamins, minerals, protei[...]
healthy. But in terms of individual vitam[...]
that a deficiency in one vitamin is almost in[...]
you have been eating a most peculiar diet. E[...]
day a diet which produces deficiency in one [...]
almost certainly produce deficiency in many, for th[...]
reason that foods which are good sources of one vitam[...]
good sources of other vitamins as well.

**Chances are you will not be aware of a vitamin
deficiency until it is quite far advanced.** Eyes and skin
show symptoms of deficiency first. If you have trouble seeing
in dim light that is night blindness which is a symptom of
vitamin A deficiency, as we have seen. If the surface of the
eye is dry, and bright lights are almost unbearable, that is a
disorder called xerophthalmia, which is also caused by a lack
of vitamin A.

The skin gets horny in someone deficient in vitamin A—
rough, dry and toad-like. Where each little hair grows on the
skin there is likely to be a horny nodule—perhaps on
shoulders, arms, chest, back and buttocks.

If you have any obvious symptoms of bad health, don't
fool yourself into thinking you can cure symptoms like those
mentioned here by eating the same old deficient diet you
have been eating and just adding some vitamins. Protein is
just as essential as the vitamins and minerals. And you must
get the protein from food—the same nutritious food which
provides the most in the way of vitamins and minerals. In the
case of vitamin A, liver is an excellent example.

An average serving of liver contains about 53,000 units of
vitamin A. Half a cup of carrots contains about 11,000 units.
The very green, fresh salad vegetables like dandelion greens
and turnip greens contain up to 15,000 units per serving.

Even allowing for generous use of butter or margarine in
cooking, most of us would not eat anything like a quarter
pound a day and that amount would supply only half the
amount of vitamin A we need. About a third of us Americans
are on reducing diets at any given time, and many reducing

...ary Sources of Vitamin A

High

...pig, sheep, calf, chicken).

...(cod, halibut, salmon, shark, sperm whale).

..., mint, kohlrabi, parsley, spinach, turnip greens,
...dandelion greens, palm oil.

Medium

Butter, cheese (except cottage), egg yolk, margarine, dried
milk, cream. White fish, eel.

Kidneys (beef, pig, sheep), liver (pork),

Mangoes, apricots, yellow melons, peaches, cherries (sour),
nectarines.

Beet greens, broccoli, endive, kale, mustard, pumpkin, sweet
potatoes, watercress, tomatoes, leek greens, chicory,
chives, collards, fennel, butterhead and romaine lettuce,
squash (acorn, butternut, hubbard), chard.

Low

Milk.

Herring, salmon, oyster, carp, clams, sardines.

Grapes, bananas, berries, (black-, goose-, rasp-, boysen-,
logan-, blue-), sweet cherries, olives, oranges, avocados,
prunes, kumquats, pineapples, plums, rhubarb, tanger-
ines, red currants.

Summer and zucchini squash, asparagus, beans (except
kidney), brussels sprouts, cabbages, leeks, peas, arti-
chokes, corn, cucumbers, lentils (dry), peppers, lettuce,
celery, cowpeas, rutabagas, okra.

Hazelnuts, peanuts, black walnuts, cashews, pecans, pis-
tachios.

Source: "Handbook of Vitamins and Hormones," by Roman J. Kutsky, Ph.D., Associate Professor of
Biology, Texas Woman's University, Denton, Texas (Van Nostrand Reinhold Co., New York,
1973, $13.50).

diets forbid the use of butter and other fa[...]
their use sharply. Other people, suffe[...]
ailments have been ordered to cut their [...]

Recently, we have been told by the Heart [...]
other experts that most of us eat too much fa[...]
advised us to cut down, for the sake of our heart a[...]
even though we may not have any current complai[...]
where are you going to get your full quota of vitamin A? Su[...]
use butter and/or margarine moderately, not in amounts like
a fourth of a pound a day.

Also get your vitamin A from leafy green vegetables and
from other bright yellow vegetables and fruits. These are the
best sources, along with liver, which is a good source of
almost anything nutritional. Sweet potatoes, squash, carrots,
tomatoes, apricots, peaches, beet greens, chard, chicory,
dandelion greens, endive, kale, mustard greens, spinach,
turnip greens also contain the vitamin.

Half a cantaloupe may contain about 3,500 units. Two whole
eggs contain about 1,140 units. The vitamin A is in the yolk
or yellow of the egg.

How often do you eat liver, carrots, salad greens,
cantaloupe, etc.? If seldom, where are you getting your
vitamin A? Is your family the "grab-a-snack-and-out-the-
door" kind? There's no vitamin A in a snack unless the snack
has been carefully chosen for its nutritional worth. Potato
chips and crackers, corn flakes, doughnuts, candy, pastry,
soft drinks, TV dinners are as devoid of vitamin A as if they
were made of cardboard. That goes for most of the other
essential nutrients as well. You must be conscious of the
importance of good diet or you are quite likely to neglect
foods in which vitamin A is abundant.

Serve liver at least once a week in some form. Serve bright
green and bright yellow vegetables like spinach and carrots
often. Serve fruits for dessert, especially the yellow ones like
peaches, cantaloupe and apricots, rather than sticky sweets.
And—need we say it?—just as added nutritional insurance,
take a daily food supplement which contains vitamin A as

ok.

butter. Isn't there a lot of vitamin A in
y ask. This is a logical question, since butter
yellow foods all contain vitamin A.

ed this up in the Department of Agriculture
k, *Composition of Foods*, where all common foods are
along with the amount of protein, vitamins and
inerals they contain. Butter and margarine contain about
3,300 units of vitamin A in 100 grams. This is about half of
what an adult needs as his recommended daily allowance of
this important vitamin. But 100 grams of butter is about one-
fourth of a pound. How many of us eat that much butter
every day? More importantly, how many of us should eat that
much butter every day?

CHAPTER 11

How Much Vitamin A Is Too Much?

IN 1973, the commissioner of the Food and Drug Administration announced new regulations which would make it impossible to sell, over the counter, any vitamin A product which contained more than 10,000 International Units of the vitamin or any vitamin D product containing more than 400 International Units of vitamin D.

The Commissioner promulgated these regulations on the basis that the vitamins in any higher potency than this would be drugs, hence he had the power to regulate them as such. They would be available in higher potencies, he announced, on prescription only. This meant, of course, that anyone wishing to take more than 10,000 units of vitamin A or more than 400 units of vitamin D at any given time would have to seek out a physician and ask him for a prescription for the higher potencies. Or the individual could simply take more than one capsule of a 10,000 unit capsule of vitamin A or a 400 unit capsule of vitamin D.

The implications of these regulations were far more

actual words they contained. Attorneys ... industry pointed out that, once such a ... ablished, it could be used to regulate all ...s of any kind in the future. If the regulations ...d to stand, the health food industry could be ... and the supplements on which many people have ...ed for years could easily become forbidden items, ...her too expensive to afford or completely unavailable if one happened to be unable to get a physician who would prescribe them.

Attorneys for the health food industry immediately took the matter to court. They have been fighting in the courts for all these past years and have now won a momentous victory for the health food movement and for everyone who takes food supplements.

On June 7, 1977, the United States Court of Appeals for the Second Circuit ruled that the 1973 regulations of the Food and Drug Administration are "invalid as arbitrary and capricious and not in accordance with law." This is a great victory for the National Nutritional Foods Association and consumer groups in their fight to protect the rights of the health food industry and the consumers of America.

Say the attorneys who fought this good fight—Bass, Ullman and Lustigman of New York City—"This has been a long and difficult struggle which proves once again what can be accomplished when we are fighting for what is right. The National Nutritional Foods Association can take just pride for the part it has played in the ever-continuing fight for freedom and justice."

In almost every article you read in the general press on the subject of vitamins, you are reminded that "some vitamins" can be toxic if consumed in large amounts. You are told to be very careful about taking vitamin A, since you may poison yourself. Usually the impression is given, deliberately, that hundreds of thousands of people are sickening and dying every year from vitamin A poisoning.

It is difficult indeed to dig out any information about

these cases of vitamin A poisoning. [text obscured]
medical literature for months and no[text obscured]
mention of anyone who was actually d[text obscured]
taken too much vitamin A, although you m[text obscured]
vague mention of this possibility.

Of course, a few bizarre cases pop up in general [text obscured]
newspapers and magazines from time to time, and [text obscured]
events, of course, are generally blown up out of proportio[text obscured]
As an example, an article in *Newsweek*, remarkable for its
malice rather than fair and honest reporting, discussed an
article which appeared in the *Journal of Nervous and Mental
Diseases*. An 18-year-old girl was admitted to a hospital
suffering from headache, blurred vision, sleep disturbances
and ringing in the ears. The optic nerve behind the eye was
swollen. "Brain tumor" decided the physician and noted that
she also had periods of mental disturbance. Upon further
inquiry, he found she had been taking vitamin A for six
months, as her doctor had told her to do in an effort to cure
her acne. The doctor had prescribed 50,000 units of vitamin
A daily. But the girl had been taking two or three times that
amount—that is, 100,000 units or 150,000 units daily. She
discontinued the vitamin and all symptoms disappeared
within a few weeks.

New Scientist for February 21, 1974 prints an almost
unbelievable report of an Englishman who killed himself
taking carrot juice and vitamin A. No one knows whether he
intended suicide or not. It seems a peculiar method of killing
oneself. This man drank, every day for many years, up to
eight pints of carrot juice, turning himself bright yellow from
the carotene pigment in the juice. In addition he took vitamin
A tablets in such extremely large amounts that, by the time of
his death, he was taking about 70,000,000 units of vitamin A.
It goes without saying that this carrot juice addict made
headlines throughout the world. Nobody takes much notice
when hundreds of thousands of people die from overdoses of
drugs, alcohol, cigarettes, sugar and other harmful things in
our modern world. But when some misguided soul takes

al food, the scientific world roars with a
you so."

k on biology, Geoffrey Bourne's *Biochemis-*
gy of Bone, stated that since 1912 more than
tamin A overdosage were reported in medical
in the entire world! This book was published some
o. Since then there have undoubtedly been more such
ses, so we were glad to get a copy of a report called *A Conspectus of Research on Vitamin A Requirements of Man* by two researchers of the Agricultural Research Service of the U. S. Department of Agriculture—Mildred S. Rodriguez and M. Isabel Irwin. These two scientists have combed medical and scientific literature and have uncovered, they say, all the reported cases of people getting too much vitamin A.

They say on page 919 of their paper, "Fifteen cases of chronic hypervitaminosis A (too much vitamin A), 12 of which occurred in the United States, have been reported." One of these people took 100,000 units of vitamin A every day for three and a half years before there was any damage to report. In another case a physician experimented with the vitamin to see how much he could take over a long period of time without trouble. He took 1,000,000 units daily for about three weeks as an experiment. In other cases people took too much vitamin A for as long as eight years before experiencing any bad effects.

What about acute poisoning—that is, enormous doses given in a short time which caused distress? The USDA scientists tell us that there is one report of 98 cases in very young children who were given doses of 300,000 to 400,000 units of vitamin A daily. In some of these, distress appeared within days, in others it took almost two years.

Five cases reported from Sweden involve infants given 7,500 to 10,000 units daily. Keep in mind that vitamin dosage is estimated by weight. That is, generally speaking, the more you weigh, the more vitamins you should have. So infants need very little compared to adults. Even so, only a few more than 100 cases of trouble were reported—in the entire world!

We asked the authors of this repo[...] covered all the cases ever reported in[...] They told us, "This covers the literatur[...]

No doubt there have been a few more ca[...] we conclude that there have been, in all of med[...] the whole world, no more than 120 to 150 case[...] getting too much vitamin A. Practically all of th[...] children or infants given too much by their parents[...] doctors—or misguided people who disregarded common sense.

In very young children there is a possibility of permanent damage from getting too much of the vitamin. For older people symptoms disappear when the massive doses are discontinued.

So **how great is the threat of getting too much vitamin A?** Every year hundreds of thousands of people are poisoned by aspirin or some other drug which can be bought casually over the counter. Countless others sicken or die from overdoses of sleeping pills or tranquilizers. A very large percentage of all patients in hospitals are suffering from "iatrogenic disease"—that is, some disorder brought on by some medication or therapy their doctors are giving them. Every drug which is advertised in medical journals must, by law, carry extensive information on possible side effects.

The effects listed are frightening indeed: nausea, vomiting, tremor, lethargy, coma, rapid heartbeat, confusion, skin eruptions, edema (swelling), constipation, menstrual irregularities, increased or decreased sex urge, jaundice, blood disease, liver disorders, cramps, dizziness, headache, rash, hives, muscle spasms, gastric irritation, blurred vision and scores of others. But over all of history only about 150 people in the world have taken too much vitamin A over long periods of time and have experienced some slight discomfort which has left them when they stopped taking the vitamin. This is the basis on which we are advised in loud warnings to beware of vitamin A.

The harm that can come from vitamin A is due to the fact

fat-soluble. That is, it is stored in body
water-soluble vitamins—vitamin C and
any excess of which is rather rapidly
and feces. So there is little or no need to
A every day, except when your doctor
it for some condition. Your body may still have
stored from last week's pill. But if you do take it every
y, the official guideline says that male adults and teenagers
need only 5,000 International Units (I.U. or units) daily.
Adult females need only 4,000 units. Infants need 1,400 and
children from 2,000 to 3,300, depending on age.

It is estimated officially that "the average American" gets
about 7,500 units of vitamin A from food: about 3,500 from
vegetables and fruits (the bright yellow and green ones);
about 2,000 units from fats, oils and dairy products (butter
and milk), about 2,000 units from meat, fish and eggs.

There is, of course, no "average American." There are
instead some 215 million people, all individual in their ways
of eating and ways of living, many with disorders which
influence their need for vitamin A. Many people eat almost
no fruits or vegetables. Those on unwise reducing diets have
been told to cut out whole milk, eggs and any fats. Many
people have given up eating meat, liver, eggs or milk out of
fear of cholesterol. Where do these folks get the recommended amount of vitamin A?

If you take mineral oil as a laxative, vitamin A is absorbed
by the oil and eliminated along with it. Certain antibiotics
also cause loss of vitamin A. Sodium benzoate (a preservative), bromobenzene, thryoxine in large concentrations, and
estrogens (the sex hormones given to women in menopause)
are destructive of vitamin A.

As we have pointed out in a number of case histories in
this book, many people become ill either because they do not
get enough vitamin A in meals or they do not properly absorb
the vitamin A they are getting. Body conditions which affect
your ability to absorb and use vitamin A are these: liver
damage, impaired absorption due to lack of bile salts, various

117

illnesses such as those which result in fa[...]
celiac disease, diabetes which makes it dif[...]
to convert carotenes (in plants) into vitar[...]
troubles and many other conditions may inte[...]
absorption of this important vitamin.

We have little information on elements in ou[...]
ment which destroy vitamin A. It seems likely that DD[...]
be destructive of the vitamin. All of us have some DDT in o[...]
fatty tissues. It seems likely that nitrates and nitrites in our
food may destroy vitamin A in our digestive tracts. Much
more research should be done in this field. It is almost
impossible to avoid these substances since they are put into
most processed meats and many other foods, and occur, as
well, in many vegetables raised with commercial nitrate
fertilizer.

So **how much vitamin A do you and your family
need?** And how much will be too much? If you eat liver once
a week, this will supply a full week's vitamin requirement and
then some—perhaps 50,000 units. If you are healthy and
have none of the disorders listed above which interfere with
vitamin A absorption, if you eat lots of bright green and
yellow vegetables plus fruits (carrots, spinach, dandelion
greens, peaches, apricots), plus eggs and whole milk, you are
getting considerable amounts of vitamin A which you can
absorb from these foods. But the very people who cannot
absorb vitamin A are the ones which have the most need for
it, for they have been getting along on very small amounts of
it for perhaps a long time. How will they make out, no matter
how much they eat of vitamin A-rich foods?

No one has ever reported any damage in an adult who is
taking up to 50,000 units of vitamin A in a food supplement
in addition to what he gets in food. Many people settle for
10,000 or 20,000 units daily to be on the safe side—as health
insurance, we say.

As long as you observe the simple precautions given here,
there is no danger at all that you will get too much vitamin A.
With infants and children, adjust the dose accordingly. And

foods that are rich in vitamin A, just
. . . king a food supplement. You need green
. . . iver, carrots and fruit for the many other
. . . contain, as well as the vitamin A.
. . . e pointed out, the water-soluble vitamins (B and
. . . y excreted if you get more than your body can use
. . . ime. There is no record of any harm from another fat-
. . . uble vitamin—vitamin E. Massive doses have been taken
without harmful effects. Vitamin D is toxic in large amounts.
Four hundred units daily is the recommended dosage. Most
milk these days is enriched with vitamin D—400 units to a
quart. Food sources of vitamin D are scarce. Nature meant us
to get this vitamin through the skin, from the action of
sunlight on the skin's oils. So spend part of every day outside,
not "suntanning" as such, but enjoying yourself in sun and
shade. You can be sure that the vitamin D will get to you. And
in winter, if you live in the north, take a vitamin D pill every
week or so, to make up for what you are not getting from the
weak, wintry sun.

Index

Pellagra, 53
Pennsylvania State University, 73
Pennsylvania, University of, 59
Pesticides, 8, 18, 23, 85
Phosphates, 23
The Pill, 86
Pittsburgh, University of, 99
Polio, 36
Pollution and Your Health, 20
Postgraduate Medicine, 60
Preservatives, chemical, 37
Proceedings of the National Academy of Sciences, 41
Prostate gland, 9, 72
Protein, 9, 18, 27, 48, 108
Psoriasis, 55, 57
Public Health Service, 6
Purdue University, 101

R

Radiation, 23, 68, 76, 79, 88
Radium, 89
Raynaud's phenomenon, 55
Respiratory tract, 9, 24, 25, 26, 87
Retinitis pigmentosa, 39
Retinoic acid, 53, 55, 56, 60, 64, 70, 91
Retinoids, 69
Rheumatic fever, 99
Rhodopsin, 38
Ringsdorf, Dr. W. M., Jr., 47
Rodriguez, Mildred S., 115
Rubiosis iritis, 45
Rutin, 50

S

Saffiotti, Dr. Umberto, 20, 76, 86, 88
Schaefer, Dr. Arnold E., 6
Schaefer, Dr. Otto, 62
Schorr, Dr. William F., 56
Schweizerische Medizinische

Wochensch.
Science, 50, 71,
Science News, 17,
Scleroderma, 55
Seborrhea, 53
Seel, Dr. David J., 100
Short-sightedness, 48
Skin, health of, 9, 52ff., 91
Smog (see "Air pollution")
Smoking, 24, 26, 33, 47, 69, 74, 75, 83, 91
Sodium benzoate, 37
Southern California, University of, 103
Southern Research Institute, Alabama, 72
Sporn, Dr. Michael B., 67
State University, Buffalo, N. Y., 38
Sterility, 99
Stilbestrol, 85, 86
Stone, Dr. Irwin, 45
Stress, 10, 74, 79
Sugar, 41, 43, 62
Sunburn, 64

T

Tea, 47
Teeth, 9
Texas, University of, 40, 106
This Week, 35
Thorium, 80
Throat, 9, 10
Thyroid gland, 37
Thyroxine, 37, 117
Tongue, 53, 54
Trichloroethylene, 88

U

Underwood, Barbara, 73
Uranium, uranium mines, 23, 79, 80
U. S. Department of Agriculture, 6, 102, 105, 111, 115

The best books on health a
nutrition are from

LARCHMONT BOOKS

___"New High-Fiber Approach to Relieving Constipation Naturally," by Adams and Murray; foreword by Sanford O. Siegal, D.O., M.D.; 320 pages, $1.95

___"Program Your Heart for Health," by Frank Murray; foreword by Michael Walczak, M.D., introduction by E. Cheraskin, M.D., D.M.D.; 368 pages, $2.95.

___"Food for Beauty," by Helena Rubinstein; revised and updated by Frank Murray, 256 pages, $1.95.

___"Eating in Eden," by Ruth Adams, 224 pages, $1.75.

___"Is Low Blood Sugar Making You a Nutritional Cripple?" by Ruth Adams and Frank Murray, 176 pages; introduction by Robert C. Atkins, M.D.; $1.75.

___"Beverages," by Adams and Murray, 288 pages, $1.75.

___"Fighting Depression," by Harvey M. Ross, M.D.; 224 pages, $1.95.

___"Health Foods," by Ruth Adams and Frank Murray, foreword by S. Marshall Fram, M.D.; 352 pages, $2.25.

___"Minerals: Kill or Cure?" by Ruth Adams and Frank Murray; foreword by Harvey M. Ross, M.D.; 368 pages, $1.95.

___"The Compleat Herbal," by Ben Charles Harris, 252 pages, $1.75.

Before ordering books from Larchmont Books, please check with local health food stores in your area. It will save postage and handling costs. If ordering by mail, please include 50¢ extra for each book for postage and handling; mail to Larchmont Books, 6 E. 43rd St., New York, N.Y. 10017.

Larchmont
Preventive Health Library

The Library will consist of the following books, [torn]
indicated. For quick reference, we have left off the full t[torn]
each book, which is "Improving Your Health with Vitamin A,[torn]
etc.

1978

1. Vitamin A
2. Niacin (Vitamin B3)
3. Vitamin C
4. Vitamin E
5. Calcium and Phosphorus
6. Zinc

1979

7. Thiamine (B1) and Riboflavin (B2)
8. Pyridoxine (B6)
9. Iodine, Iron and Magnesium
10. Sodium and Potassium
11. Copper, Chromium and Selenium
12. Vitamin B12 and Folic Acid

1980

13. Vitamin D and Vitamin K
14. Pantothenic Acid
15. Biotin, Choline, Inositol and PABA
16. Protein and Amino Acids
17. Natural Foods
18. Other Trace Minerals